LECTURE NOTES ON

NEON

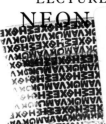

LECTURE NOTES ON
NEONATOLOGY

G.M.GANDY
MD MB BS MRCP DCH

N.R.C.ROBERTON
MA MB BChir FRCP

both of
The Department of Paediatrics
Rosie Maternity Hospital, Cambridge

BLACKWELL SCIENTIFIC PUBLICATIONS

OXFORD LONDON EDINBURGH

BOSTON PALO ALTO MELBOURNE

First published 1987

Set by Setrite Typesetters Ltd
Hong Kong
Printed and bound at
Alden Press Ltd, Oxford

DISTRIBUTORS

USA
  Year Book Medical Publishers
  35 East Wacker Drive
  Chicago, Illinois 60601
Canada
  The C.V. Mosby Company
  5240 Finch Avenue East
  Scarborough, Ontario

Australia
  Blackwell Scientific Publications
  (Australia) Pty Ltd
  107 Barry Street
  Carlton, Victoria 3053

British Library
Cataloguing in Publication Data

Gandy, Gillian M.
  Lecture notes on neonatology.
  1. Infants (Newborn) — Diseases
  I. Title   II. Roberton, N.R.C.
  618.92'01   RJ254

ISBN 0-632-00992-6

Contents

Preface

Six hundred thousand babies are born each year in England and Wales and during the first day, week and month of their lives, they are statistically at greater risk of serious illness or death than at any other time in childhood. The care of these babies occupies a large part of the time of many doctors, nurses and midwives working in neonatal units, postnatal wards and sometimes also at home.

Although there are large reference books for the full-time neonatal specialist, and in recent years a proliferation of manuals on how to look after a very ill, ventilated 1000 g baby, there is also a need for a brief general outline of the problems of the newborn baby, both full-term, small for dates and premature.

This book has been written to fulfil that need, and we have laid it out in a way which will enable the reader to find easily the answers to specific subjects such as the normal preterm and small for dates baby, or how to examine or feed entirely normal fullterm babies. We have also touched on perinatal bereavement, as well as the follow-up of the survivors of extreme prematurity.

In addition, we have tried to cover the common neonatal illnesses in a simple, system-orientated way. Throughout we have referred to the baby as 'he'. This is not sexist, merely a tacit recognition that the neonatal male is the weaker sex, and much more likely to suffer from the conditions discussed in the text.

This book will be useful for medical, nursing and midwifery students, and will also be of value to midwives, obstetricians, and GPs who are involved in neonatal care, particularly with the excellent modern trend to devolve the care of the bigger preterm baby and the normal growth-retarded baby onto the postnatal ward and into the home.

Finally we hope that it will be of value to everyone involved in maternity care who needs some understanding of the serious diseases which affect very preterm infants, and will enable them to talk sensibly about these problems to the baby's parents.

GMG, NRCR
Cambridge

Acknowledgments

Many people, too many to name, have helped in the preparation of this book by doing our work whilst we have been hunched over our notes or word processor. We would, however, particularly like to thank Dr N.D. Barnes who read Chapters 10 and 23 and advised on their content; Professor Fergus McCartney was very helpful with his advice for Chapter 17. We are very grateful to Chris Green and the Department of Medical Illustration at Addenbrooke's for their help with the preparation of the illustrations. NRCR is totally indebted to his wife who typed his part of the manuscript (several times!)

Finally we are very grateful to all the editorial staff at Blackwell Scientific Publications for their help in the production of the work, and particularly to Peter Saugman for his good natured and persistent chivvying as the gestation of this work went way past term.

GMG, NRCR
Cambridge

Abbreviations

ACD	acid citrate dextrose (anti-coagulant)	GA	gestational age
ACTH	adrenocorticotrophic hormone	GFR	glomerular filtration rate
AD	autosomal dominant	GI	gastro-intestinal
ADH	antidiuretic hormone	GLH	germinal layer haemorrhage
AP	anterior/posterior	HDN	haemolytic disease of the newborn
APTT	activated partial thromboplastin time	HIE	hypoxic ischaemic encephalopathy
AR	autosomal recessive	HMD	hyaline membrane disease
AS	aortic stenosis	IDM	infants of diabetic mothers
ASD	atrial septal defect	IMV	intermittent mandatory ventilation
ATN	acute tubular necrosis		
AV	atrioventricular	IPPV	intermittent positive pressure ventilation
BP	blood pressure		
BPD	bronchopulmonary dysplasia	IRT	immunoreactive trypsin
CAH	congenital adrenal hyperplasia	IVH	intraventricular haemorrhage
CBF	cerebral blood flow	IUGR	intra-uterine growth retardation
CDH	congenital dislocation of the hips		
		JVP	jugular venous pressure
CMV	cytomegalovirus	LB	live births
CNS	central nervous system	LBW	low birthweight
CPAP	continuous positive airway pressure	L:S	lecithin: sphingomyelin
		MCT	medium chain triglyceride
CPD	citrate phosphate dextrose (anti-coagulant)	MI	mitral incompetence
		NEC	necrotizing enterocolitis
CPIP	chronic pulmonary insufficiency of prematurity	NNICU	neonatal intensive care unit
		NNM	neonatal mortality
CSF	cerebrospinal fluid	NNU	neonatal unit
CT	computerized tomography	NTD	neural tube defect
CVP	central venous pressure	OFC	occipito-frontal head circumference
CVS	cardiovascular system		
CXR	chest X-ray	OPCS	Office of Population Censuses & Surveys
DBM	'drip' breast milk		
DIC	disseminated intravascular coagulation	PCV	packed cell volume
		PDA	patent ductus arteriosus
DPL	dipalmitoyl lecithin	PEEP	positive end expiratory pressure
EBM	expressed breast milk		
ECF	extracellular fluid	PFC	persistent fetal circulation
ECG	electrocardiogram	PGE	prostaglandin E
EEG	electroencephalogram	PIE	pulmonary interstitial emphysema
ETT	exercise tolerance test		
FRC	functional residual capacity	PKU	phenlyketonuria

PNM	perinatal mortality	TAPVD	total anomalous pulmonary venous drainage
PNW	postnatal ward		
PPF	plasma protein fraction	TEV	talipes equino-varus
PS	pulmonary stenosis	THAM	tris-hydroxymethylamino-methane
PT	prothombin		
PVH	periventricular haemorrhage	TOF	tracheo-oesophageal fistula
PVL	periventricular leucomalacia	TPN	total parenteral nutrition
RDS	respiratory distress syndrome	TSH	thyroid stimulating hormone
REM	rapid eye movement	TTN	transient tachypnoea of the newborn
RLF	retrolental fibroplasia		
ROP	retinopathy of prematurity	UAC	umbilical artery catheter
RR	respiratory rate	UTI	urinary tract infection
SEH	subependymal haemorrhage	UVC	umbilical venous catheter
SFD	small for dates	VLBW	very low birthweight
SMA	synthetic milk adapted	VSD	ventricular septal defect

Section I

Chapter 1
Introduction

The care of the newborn infant has excited the attention and the imagination of physicians since before the time of Christ, but it was only about 100 years ago, starting in France with Tarnier and Budin at the Paris Maternity Hospital, Porte Royale, that concerted efforts were made to provide facilities for the care of low birthweight infants. The development of incubators in Paris in the 1880s, commercialized by Couney at exhibitions in Berlin, Paris and London in the 1890s, was the first comparatively widespread introduction of technology into neonatal care, although William Smellie had described laryngeal intubation in 1752, and various attempts at ventilation were published in the latter part of that century.

Following the pioneering efforts of Tarnier, Budin and Couney special care baby units were built in many centres in North America and continental Europe in the first half of the twentieth century, yet neonatal care in Britain remained in the doldrums. The conspicuous and notable exception to this generalization was Dr Mary Crosse who established a nursery for preterm babies in the Sorrento Hospital in Birmingham in 1931. Despite her pioneering efforts half a century ago, it is only in the last 20 years that neonatal care has become a major preoccupation of British paediatricians.

In the immediate post-war years some interest in neonatal medicine was catalysed by an understanding of the treatment of rhesus haemolytic disease, by the pioeering work of paediatricians like Blackfan and Silverman on the maintenance of an adequate thermal environment for low birthweight infants, and most of all by the catastrophic outbreaks in the 1940s and 1950s of iatrogenic disease in the neonate, in particular retinopathy of prematurity (ROP) (p.317).

Concurrently with this increasing clinical awareness, two major advances in medical science furthered the cause of the sick neonate. Firstly, an increasing number of distinguished physiologists, stimulated by Barron in the USA and by Sir Joseph Barcroft in Cambridge, began to unravel the complexities of fetal, and in particular, neonatal physiology. Secondly, vast improvements in medical laboratory technology enabled sophisticated biochemical, haematological, immunological and blood gas investigations to be carried out on small enough

3

samples of blood for intensive laboratory monitoring of the sick low birthweight infant without the baby being exsanguinated within 24 hours of delivery. When Dr Wilfrid Payne announced (Acharya and Payne, 1965) that he could do seventeen biochemical investigations on 1.3 ml of neonatal blood, the age of intensive neonatal monitoring had dawned.

The possibility of converting these physiological and technical advances into clinical practice was fostered in Britain by two Government reports. In 1961, the then Ministry of Health published *Prevention of Prematurity and the Care of Premature Infants* (Ministry of Health, 1961), which recommended the establishment of special care nurseries, and recommended that they should have six cots for every 1000 births in the hospital. In 1971 the Department of Health and Social Security backed up these recommendations with the *Report of the Expert Group on Special Care for Babies* (Sheldon Report, DHSS, 1971) which, in addition, gave guidelines on the indications for admission to neonatal units and staffing levels for both special and intensive care. These reports, coupled with an increased awareness among the general public as well as paediatricians, obstetricians, midwives and administrators, of the benefits of proper care being available for low birthweight infants from the moment of birth, meant that by the mid-1970s, no maternity unit worth its salt was without some form of special care baby unit.

Although the facilities in many parts of Britain for neonatal intensive care — as opposed to special care — are still far from ideal, considerable improvements have occurred in neonatal intensive care in the last decade. As a result, a woman who reaches 30 weeks gestation, and/or can produce a normally formed baby weighing more than 1250—1300 g will almost certainly have a neurologically intact surviving baby. At less than 30 weeks gestation, the survival rate is steadily improving, and it is now clear that the commonly accepted definition of viability (28 weeks of gestation) is no longer tenable, since many infants survive at 26 weeks of gestation or less. It is with this group of infants at gestations of 26—30 weeks who often have severe respiratory disease (p.129), sepsis (p.172), or the most feared complication of all, periventricular haemorrhage (p.215), and who are most at risk from the permanently disabling complications of cerebral palsy and blindness from ROP, that modern neonatal intensive care is most concerned.

Nevertheless, a large component of neonatal medicine is still to do with the care of the normal baby, both term and low birthweight.

This book is an attempt to introduce the student to both these aspects of neonatal care.

References

Acharya, P.T. & Payne, W.W. (1965) Blood chemistry of normal full term infants in the first 48 hours of life. *Archives of Diseases in Childhood* **40**, 430–5.

Department of Health & Social Security (1971) *Report of the Expert Group on Special Care Babies* (Reports on Public Health and Medical Subjects No. 127). HMSO, London.

Ministry of Health (1961) *Prevention of Prematurity and the Care of Premature Infants.* HMSO, London.

Chapter 2
Definitions, Statistics and Epidemiology

Definitions (Fig. 2.1)

Gestation

Prematurity

A neonate, irrespective of birthweight, born before 37 weeks of pregnancy (i.e. <259 days) timed from the first day of the last menstrual period.

Term

A baby born between the 37th and 42nd weeks of pregnancy (i.e. 259–294 days).

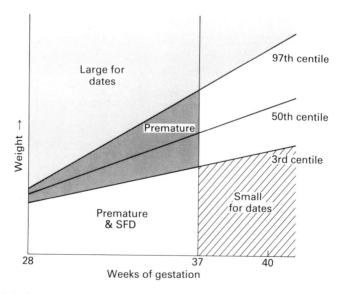

Fig. 2.1. Categories of newborn babies.

6

Postmature

A neonate irrespective of birthweight born after the 42nd week of gestation (i.e. >294 days).

Birthweight

Low birthweight (LBW)

This comprises the 6–7% of all infants weighing ≤2.5 kg at birth. Many premature neonates as defined above weigh more than this; conversely, about one-third of infants weighing ≤2.5 kg at birth are more than 37 weeks gestation.

Very low birthweight (VLBW)

Although there is no internationally accepted definition of such babies, by common consent this term applies to the 0.8–1.5% of all neonates weighing <1.5 kg at birth. A large proportion of all serious illness, and two-thirds of all non-malformation neonatal deaths occur in this group of infants. About one-third of this group weigh <1.0 kg at birth and are an ever-increasing problem in neonatal care.

Small for dates (SFD)

Babies whose birthweight falls below some predetermined cut-off point at a given gestational age (GA) (Fig. 2.1). Some paediatricians choose the third centile, others the fifth centile, and others two standard deviations below the normal birthweight for the gestation (Table 2.1). SFD infants can be either premature, fullterm or postmature (Fig. 2.1).

Table 2.1. Weight criteria for *SFD* babies as used in the Rosie Maternity Hospital, Cambridge. (After Usher & McLean 1969.)

GA (weeks)	−2 SD for birthweight
36	1890
37	2120
38	2335
39	2500
40	2615
41	2550
42	2510

Large for dates

A baby whose birthweight lies above some predetermined cut-off point at a given GA, usually above the 97th centile (Fig. 2.1).

Mortality rates

Stillbirth/stillbirth rate

An infant born dead on or after the 28th week of gestation (i.e. 196 days). The stillbirth rate is expressed per 1000 total births (i.e. live births plus stillbirths). In 1984 the rate for England and Wales was 5.7/1000 births.

Neonatal death/neonatal mortality rate

An infant born alive at any gestation (including those born at <28 weeks) who dies within 28 days of delivery. By convention it is usually divided into early neonatal deaths — those dying in the first 7 days, and late neonatal deaths — those dying between the 8th and 28th day. The mortality rate is expressed per 1000 LB. In 1984 in England and Wales, the early neonatal mortality was 4.4/1000 LB and the late neonatal mortality was 1.1/1000 LB, with a total neonatal mortality of 5.5/1000 LB. The fall in neonatal mortality in England and Wales over the last half century is shown in Fig. 2.2.

Perinatal death/perinatal mortality rate

This is the stillbirth rate plus the early neonatal mortality rate expressed per 1000 births. In 1984 in England and Wales it was 10.1/1000 births. The fall in perinatal mortality in the last half century is also shown in Fig. 2.2.

Infant mortality

This is the overall death rate in babies under the age of 1 year, including neonatal deaths. In 1984 the infant mortality in England and Wales was 9.5/1000 LB. By subtracting the total neonatal mortality of 5.5/1000 LB this leaves a mortality rate of 4.0/1000 for infants aged 29–365 days.

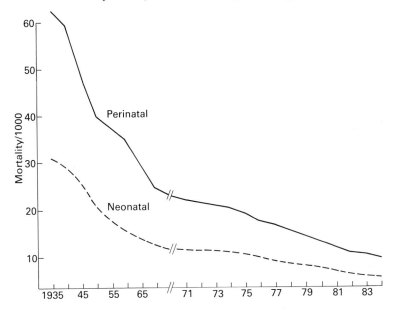

Fig. 2.2. Neonatal and perinatal mortality in England and Wales 1935–84.

Causes of perinatal death

Despite continuing attempts to obtain post-mortem examination on all stillbirths and neonatal deaths, it is surprisingly difficult to obtain interpretable data about the cause of stillbirths in particular.

In the 1980s, despite selective termination of many malformed infants detected early in pregnancy by ultrasound or amniotic fluid analysis, it is clear that lethal malformations are still responsible for a large proportion of stillbirths (Table 2.2).

Once malformations are excluded from Table 2.2, however, it is clear that a large number of stillbirths are either completely unexplained or are associated in some vague, non-specific way with a maternal illness. The latter could cause fetal asphyxia by, for example, reduced placental blood flow or the abnormal vascularity in the placenta associated with maternal toxaemia.

Similar, but less severe, problems occur when attempting to get some epidemiological overview of causes of neonatal death. The returns from the Office of Population Censuses and Surveys (OPCS) (formerly the Registrar General) contain diagnostic criteria for causes of death which do not make clinical sense. These include attributing a

Chapter 2

Table 2.2. Causes of stillbirth.

	Scottish Perinatal Mortality Survey 1977 (McIlwaine et al. 1979)	University of Washington 1979–81 (Mueller et al. 1983)	Cambridge Maternity Hospital 1978–84 (unpubl.)
Stillbirth (unexplained, no maternal illness)	177 (35%)		70 (42%)
Antepartum haemorrhage (primarily abruptio placentae)	51 (10%)	26 (37%)	25 (15%)
Maternal illness (including toxaemia)	69 (14%)		7 (4%)
Intrapartum stillbirth	96 (19%)		8 (5%)
Congenital malformation	101 (20%)	23 (32%)	47 (28%)
Twin	*	5	5
Rhesus	8	2	1
Other	2	17[†] (24%)	2

*Excluded from analysis.
[†]Attributed primarily to chorioamnionitis.

neonatal death to some maternal complication of pregnancy, or just to low birthweight, when in fact the baby probably died of respiratory distress syndrome (RDS, p.129) or periventricular haemorrhage (PVH, p.215). As with the data on stillbirths, the proportion of deaths due to individual diagnoses in large national data collection systems is very different from that found in small, carefully analysed local studies (Table 2.3). Nationally, over 50% of deaths are attributed to asphyxia, low birthweight (unspecified), or other diagnoses, compared with 20% in Cambridge, suggesting a poorer level of diagnostic accuracy in the OPCS figures.

One other reason for this disparity is that it may often be difficult to explain the cause of a baby's death accurately. For example, most infants who die from RDS are probably killed by an associated PVH — since without this complication survival in RDS is now the rule (Table 2.4). Yet, which of these two diagnoses, RDS or PVH, should be coded as the primary cause of death, and thus included in the statistics?

Table 2.3. Causes of neonatal death. Comparison of national and local data (the figures in brackets are the percentage of all neonatal deaths).

	RDS	Malformations*	Infection	Asphyxia	Low birthweight (unspecified)	Other	Total
Neonatal deaths, Cambridge Maternity Hospital, 1982–85							
≤1.5 kg	40 (29.2%)	10 (7.3%)	11 (8.0%)	1	7 (5.1%)	11[†] (8.0%)	80 (58.4%)
1.5–2.5 kg	2	14 (10.2%)	3 (2.2%)	—	—	2[†]	21 (15.3%)
>2.5 kg	—	25 (18.2%)	3 (2.2%)	7 (5.1%)	—	1	36 (26.2%)
Neonatal deaths, England and Wales, 1983 (OPCS)							
≤1.5 kg	399 (11.5%)	154 (4.4%)	41 (1.2%)	133 (3.8%)	372 (10.7%)	469[††] (13.5%)	1568 (45.1%)
1.5–2.5 kg	108 (3.1%)	351 (10.1%)	37 (1.1%)	100 (2.9%)	9	257 (7.4%)	754 (21.7%)
>2.5 kg	21 (0.6%)	596 (17.2%)	43 (1.2%)	243 (7.0%)	8	263 (7.6%)	1153 (33.2%)

*Includes lethal metabolic errors and congenital tumours.
[†]Includes 6 (5<1.5 kg) with pulmonary hypoplasia after prolonged membrane rupture.
[††]Includes 132 attributed to other respiratory disease and 109 to fetal and neonatal haemorrhage (? PVH).

Table 2.4. Causes of death in babies ≤1.5 kg, 1982–85, Cambridge Maternity Hospital.

Cause of death	Number of deaths
RDS plus intracranial bleed	32
RDS plus airleak	5
RDS plus pulmonary haemorrhage	2
RDS solo	1
Lethal malformations	10
Septicaemia	9
Extreme prematurity (<26 weeks)	6
Pulmonary hypoplasia	5
Miscellaneous	7

Interpretation of perinatal statistics

For many years neonatal and perinatal mortality figures from different countries have been compared, as have similar data from different health authorities, towns and teaching hospitals. On the basis of the position in the mortality league table, various judgements have been made about the standards of perinatal care in these services. There are three major reasons why it is a totally unacceptable practice to use the raw neonatal or perinatal mortality data in this way:

1 There is considerable variation between populations in the percentage of babies weighing less that 2.5 kg at birth (Table 2.5). Since the majority of neonatal deaths, particularly those not due to lethal malformations, occur in these infants, these variations are likely to have much more influence on the neonatal mortality than the standards of care available locally.

2 The problem with allowing for the number of LBW infants included in the data is particularly important when discussing VLBW infants. There is a wide unit-to-unit and district-to-district variation in the registration practice for such infants — both stillbirths and neonatal deaths, particularly those weighing less that 800 g and of 24–27 weeks gestation. Since a very large proportion of the neonatal mortality is now in these infants, if they are called abortions and excluded from the perinatal statistics, it will have a marked effect on the comparability of neonatal and perinatal mortality data.

3 The malformation rate is different in different communities — that for anencephaly showing a particularly marked variation (Fig. 2.3). Yet this single condition alone could account for Ireland having a perinatal mortality of 3.5/1000 births worse than Finland and Japan.

Table 2.5.   Incidence of low birthweight (≤2.5 kg) in different countries.

Country	Percentage incidence
India	28.0
Malaysia	16.8
Phillipines	14.2
Cuba	10.8
Hungary	10.8
Singapore	7.4
England	6.7
USA	6.0
Austria	5.7
Japan	5.3
Sweden	3.9

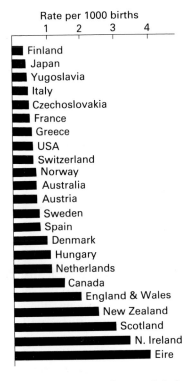

Fig. 2.3. Incidence (per 1000 total births) of anencephaly in various countries (From Chalmers & MacFarlance, 1980.)

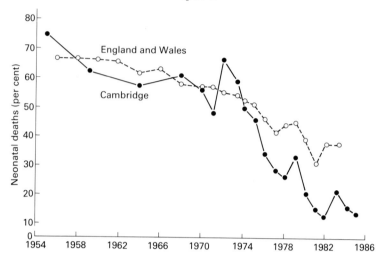

Fig. 2.4. Neonatal mortality 1000–1500 g birthweight.

Table 2.6. Perinatal and neonatal mortality, Cambridge Maternity Hospital 1977–85 (excluding lethal malformations and all deaths ≤1.0 kg birthweight).

Year	PNM/1000 deliveries	NNM/1000 LB
1977	6.8	2.7
1978	7.1	2.6
1979	7.1	2.2
1980	5.8	2.5
1981	5.0	1.4
1982	4.8	2.1
1983	4.4	2.2
1984	4.0	2.3
1985	3.6	1.4

Bearing these factors in mind, it is clear that perinatal statistics need very careful interpretation. One effective and justifiable way of looking at mortality data is to consider just those infants in a 500 g birthweight cohort. Figure 2.4 shows such data for infants weighing 1.0–1.5 kg, where, as can be seen, the impact of neonatal intensive care from the early 1970s onwards has had a marked effect on reducing neonatal mortality both on the national and local scene.

Another widely-used technique, which makes region-to-region comparisons of neonatal mortality and perinatal mortality more acceptable, is to remove all infants with lethal malformations from the data, and to restrict the analysis to infants with a birthweight greater than 1.0 kg. When this is done (Table 2.6) it can be seen that although there is a trend towards reducing the incidence of stillbirth and neonatal death, there remains a hard core of about 4/1000 perinatal deaths which is proving very difficult to eradicate.

References

Chalmers, I. & MacFarlane, A. (1980) Interpretation of statistics. In *Topics in Perinatal Medicine*, B.A. Wharton (ed.), Pitman Medical, London, pp. 1–11.

MacIlwaine, G.M., Howat, R.C.L., Dunn F. & McNaughton M.C. (1979), *Scotland 1977. Perinatal Mortality Survey*. Dept. of Obstetrics and Gynaecology, University of Glasgow.

Mueller, R.F., Sybert, V.P., Johnson, J., Brown, Z.A. & Chen, W.J. (1983) Evaluation of a protocol for post-mortem examination of stillbirths. *New England Journal of Medicine* **309**, 586–90.

Usher, R.H. & McLean, F.H. (1969). Intrauterine growth of liveborn Caucasian infants at sea level: standards obtained from measurements in 7 dimensions of infants born between 25 and 44 weeks gestation. *Journal of Pediatrics* **74**, 901–10.

Further reading

Mutch, L.M.M. (1986) Neonatal epidemiology. In *Textbook of Neonatology*, N.R.C. Roberton (ed.), Churchill Livingstone, Edinburgh. pp. 3–19.

Chapter 3
Mother–Child Interaction

In the last 10 years a wealth of scientific evidence has emphasized the importance of encouraging parent–child contact in the early neonatal period. This has given rise to the concept of 'bonding' or 'attachment', which is basically the process by which the mother and her newborn baby get to know, and learn to love, each other.

Term babies

The seminal study on this subject was that of Marshall Klaus and John Kennell in Cleveland, USA (1982). They studied a group of 28 newborn babies and their poor, largely unmarried, inner-city, black mothers. Half of the mothers had the routine nursery access to their babies: during any 24 hour period they had them for only 20–30 minutes every 4 hours for feeding. The other group had 1 hour alone with their baby within 3 hours of delivery, and an additional 5 hours per day with their baby in the postnatal ward (PNW) over and above the contact for feeding described above. On follow-up, the mothers with extended contact were:

1 More caring and comforting to their babies during routine paediatric physical examination in the first year.
2 More likely to talk to their babies rather than order them about.
3 More confident in their ability to care for and handle their babies.

  It has been said that this study of poor, single, black mothers in American hospitals has little relevance to British maternity hospitals where mothers normally have much more contact with their newborn infants. However, a succession of subsequent studies both in Europe and America on term infants, or slightly premature infants in the 2.0–2.5 kg birthweight range, have all come to the same conclusion. This is, that the more contact the mother has with her baby in the neonatal period, the *less likely* it is that there will be problems during infancy with:

1 Establishing and maintaining breast-feeding.
2 Feeding problems in general, including failure to thrive.
3 Difficult baby behaviour such as persistent crying, irritability or attention-seeking.

No study of term babies has shown any benefits at all from *increased* mother—child separation!

One specific point to emphasize is the importance of letting the mother and baby be together during the first hour after delivery. In the first hour of life, newborn babies are particularly wide-eyed, wide awake and appealing, and their mothers should be given the opportunity to enjoy them while they are like that; one of the major determinants of successful long-term lactation is whether or not an infant suckles at the breast during the first hour. However, there is no need to invoke the dubious concept that this critical and sensitive period is the only time when attachment can take place — as occurs in animals — in order to encourage mother—baby contact during this time.

Preterm babies

With preterm babies weighing less than 1.8 kg, and in particular those weighing less than 1.2 kg, who are likely to spend several weeks or months in a neonatal unit (NNU), often undergoing intensive care, the problems of parent—baby attachment are even greater. Studies of mother and parent—baby interaction in this LBW group consistently highlight three important points:

1 Mothers find it acutely disturbing to be separated from their preterm neonates, and the more intensive the care applied to their babies, in general, the more disturbing it becomes.

2 When a mother takes home a baby who has spent a long time in a neonatal intensive care unit, it takes her a long time to 'get to know' him; such babies are much more likely than term babies to pose feeding and behavioural problems, or to suffer from failure to thrive and child-abuse during infancy.

3 The more efforts that are made to bring mothers into the neonatal intensive care unit (NNICU) and involve them in the care of their babies, the more the above problems are mitigated, though they can never be completely avoided. Visiting and staying in an NNICU provokes considerable maternal anxiety, but most mothers prefer to cope with this rather than be unable to visit their baby.

The routines which should be instituted to mitigate the problems faced by the mothers of VLBW infants in NNICUs include the following:

1 Senior members of the nursing or medical staff may need to spend a lot of time explaining to the parents what is happening to their baby, and to be prepared to repeat what they have said. Under the extreme

stress of having their baby admitted to a NNICU, few parents retain much of what is said to them during the first, or even second and third, consultations.

2 Let parents see their baby for a short time on the labour ward if he has to be admitted to the NNICU immediately after birth, and explain to them why the admission is necessary.

3 Thereafter get the parents, and particularly the father, up to the NNICU as soon as possible to see the baby.

4 Allow unrestricted 24-hour access to the unit for parents throughout their baby's stay.

5 Allow the parents into the unit without asking them to put on gowns or masks, but give them careful instructions about handwashing. Encourage them to stroke, touch and talk to their critically ill baby even if he is receiving IPPV, and to get involved subsequently by cuddling, feeding and changing him even if he still requires oxygen.

6 Allow unrestricted access for grandparents and siblings, and have a liberal approach to visiting by other family members.

7 Give the mother a photograph of her baby to keep on her beside table, particularly if she is unlikely to be able to get to see the baby either because she is in another hospital or because she is too ill to come from another part of the maternity hospital to the NNICU.

8 Give all parents a small handbook which explains in non-technical language precisely what happens on the NNICU.

9 Encourage the mother to provide expressed breast milk for her own baby with instructions on how to use electrical breast pumps if necessary.

10 Move the mothers of neonatal transfers with their babies, and admit them to the postnatal ward of the maternity hospital or to one of the NNICU's mother and baby rooms.

11 Allow parents to stay with and hold their dying infants, or to take infants with inoperable malformations home for terminal care (see Chapter 32).

Reference

Klaus, M.H. & Kennell, J.H. (1982) *Parent Infant Bonding*, 2nd edn. C.V. Mosby Company, St. Louis.

Further reading

Davis, J.A., Richards, M.P.M. & Roberton, N.R.C. (1983) *Parent Baby Attachment in Premature Infants*. Croom Helm, Beckenham.

Chapter 4
Talking to parents

Introduction

During pregnancy a mother builds up a relationship with her obstetric attendants. After delivery she is suddenly confronted by individuals whose prime interest lies in the new arrival. Lack of communication leads to bewildered, frightened and resentful parents; phrases like 'they never tell you anything' are still all too common. This chapter sets out some guidelines and highlights some problem areas.

Principles

1 Obtain basic information about the mother's obstetric and medical history either from the notes or by discussion with others who are familiar with her problems. Find out if there are any complicated social factors; knowledge of the parents' occupation and social background can be extremely helpful in gauging the level at which to pitch conversations. The GP may be an invaluable source of information.

2 Introduce yourself and engage in some preliminary pleasantries to get the 'feel' of the situation. Ask the parents what they know or have been told about the baby already.

3 Try to talk *with* parents and not at them; it is helpful if you are all on the same level, whether it be standing up or preferably sitting. Also remember to *look* at them during the conversation; it is amazing how often this simple principle is forgotten. Valuable visual clues can often be gained on both sides.

4 There are seldom complaints about giving too much information. One need not share every anxiety with the parents, but generally more harm is done by withholding information than by giving it.

5 Try to ensure consistency. One common complaint from parents (and patients) is that they are told different things by different people. Often this is not strictly true, but the important thing is that different messages have got through. This problem can be mitigated, to some extent, by:

a Reducing the number of would-be advisors.

b Ensuring adequate communication between other hospital staff.

c Remembering to tell the GP, community midwife or health visitor what has been said.

6 Having explained the baby's condition, always ask the parents if they have any questions, or promise to return when they have had time to think; they seldom take in what is said on the first occasion, so be prepared to repeat yourself.

7 The mother wants to hear that her baby is perfect in every way; any suggestion to the contrary is bound to produce considerable distress. Mothers are often emotionally very labile after delivery and need constant reassurance. It is all too easy to be obsessed by the *physical* care for the infant and fail to realize how much emotional support is needed in the case of a sick or abnormal baby.

Where and when to talk to parents

Pre-delivery

Talking to the mother before delivery may be very helpful if any postnatal problems are anticipated.

Labour ward

An almost universal question after delivery is 'is he alright?' Most babies behave in the approved manner, but a reassuring word to an anxious couple may make all the difference. There are a few occasions when it is mandatory to talk to the parents soon after birth.

1 Following prolonged or difficult resuscitation, tell them about it and try to answer any questions.

2 A small but otherwise well baby (<1.8 kg) will almost certainly go to the neonatal unit, but always show him to the parents; let them hold him and explain what is involved.

3 It is equally essential to allow the parents to have a glimpse of a sick baby, even if on a ventilator. Tell them that they can soon come to see him.

4 If there is an obvious major malformation, e.g. hare lip, cleft palate, talipes, spina bifida, anal atresia or ambiguous genitalia, the parents will need some information immediately, although this must be non-committal until the lesion can be more carefully examined.

Postnatal ward

Talking to parents of normal fullterm babies is covered in Chapter 7. Other situations are:

1 The small or preterm baby who is in hospital with his mother for 2 weeks or more. It is all too easy to forget these infants; the mother is often glad to have a chat about his progress or any problems.

2 The baby who becomes ill on the PNW or needs transfer to the NNU. This is an extremely alarming experience for the mother. Always explain what is happening and return as soon as possible after the problem has been more clearly defined; encourage her to come to the NNU.

The neonatal unit

The general management of the family of a baby in an NNU is outlined in Chapter 3. The sight and sounds of an intensive care unit with rows of monitors, flashing lights, equipment and alarms sounding off are terrifying to the mother of a newly-born baby who appears to be utterly lost in a maze of wires and tubes.

The parents will want to know why they produced a small or sickly infant; whether he will grow and develop normally. Tell them what to expect, reassure them that their feelings of inadequacy are natural. Let them air their feelings and try to alleviate worries about older siblings at home, father's time off work or the cost of travel.

Explain the nature of the baby's illness, treatment and likely outcome; use simple diagrams to illustrate problems. Sick preterm infants often have a stormy course over the first few days and can rapidly deteriorate, only to recover within minutes; warn them about these see-saw cycles so that they are not too disappointed when the next setback occurs. Be reasonably optimistic unless the infant is really desperately sick. Demonstrate and explain the function of all the attached equipment, e.g. catheters, endotracheal and nasogastric tubes, electrodes, monitors and ventilators.

Some specific situations

Intraventricular haemorrhage

Mention of any lesion connected with the brain will almost certainly produce anxiety. It is probably unnecessary to mention a small germinal layer or intraventricular haemorrhage (Chapter 18) because such lesions can occur in up to 40% of infants <1.5 kg without apparent deleterious effects. In the case of a massive periventricular haemorrhage something should probably be said. Phrases like 'cerebral haemorrhage' and 'brain damage' are almost guaranteed to strike terror into the parents' hearts; great tact is needed to explain the nature and possible sequelae of such lesions.

Chronic illness in the newborn

Some small infants take a long time to be weaned off the ventilator because of chronic lung disease or recurrent apnoea (Chapter 15). Many weeks may pass when the baby makes little or no progress. Parents can become very depressed by the long illness, wondering if they will ever have their infant home. This requires repeated and prolonged discussions; parent support groups may be very valuable.

Congenital malformations

To produce a baby with some major defect is a devastating blow to the parents. The stages of reaction through which they commonly pass (Fig. 4.1) are:

1 Shock accompanied by much crying and helplessness.

2 Denial and a wish to escape from the problem.

3 Sadness, anger and resentment which may encompass a reluctance to accept the baby.

4 Some degree of equilibrium is established with increasing confidence in the ability to cope, but still intermingled with periods of sadness.

5 Finally, in a stage of reorganization and adaptation, the parents

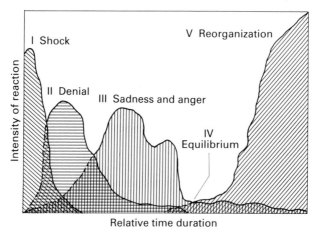

Fig. 4.1. Stages of parents' emotional reactions. (From Drosar *et al.*, 1975.)

begin to deal with the situation in a practical way and accept the baby for what he is.

The manner and speed of progress through these grief reactions is very variable and may depend on the nature of the malformation. Is it visible? Can it be treated? Does it affect the brain? Are there other abnormalities? Will the baby die? Could it happen again? The initial concern is usually greater with visible malformations. Lesions that involve the CNS or genitalia are likely to lead to the most turmoil and are the hardest to come to terms with.

General principles for talking about a malformed baby

1 Always see both parents together if at all possible, and remember that it is the manner of telling rather than the actual words which make an indelible impression.
2 Never attempt to hide him; an imagined abnormality is usually much worse than the reality. Even mothers of anencephalics are glad to have seen the baby. Failure to have a proper image may drastically interfere with the mourning process.
3 Take a photograph of the baby if he is stillborn or dies.
4 Demonstrate and explain the abnormality, but be at pains to highlight the favourable and positive points.
5 Outline the treatment if any is indicated. Answering questions about the future may take many sessions.
6 Explaining the cause of an abnormality may be difficult since it is often unknown. Bring up the subject so that the parents can express any guilt feelings but reassure them that it is not their fault.
7 Support. Unless the abnormality is life-threatening the baby should remain with his mother; she needs repeated visits by staff and plenty of opportunity to express her feelings. Always inform the GP who probably has a wide knowledge of the family. There are now many support groups for parents of malformed babies, and details of these should be available.
8 Will it happen again? This question is almost bound to come up at some point; give advice and/or arrange genetic counselling.

Down's syndrome

There is no doubt that parents should be given the diagnosis relatively early and if they suspect some abnormal features they must be told immediately. Informing unsuspecting parents that they have a Down's baby is best done by a senior staff member. The following guidelines may be helpful:

1 Make sure of the diagnosis; clinical features are usually sufficient. You may have to see the baby while he is in the nursery away from the mother.

2 Arrange to see the parents together (e.g. when the father comes to visit), and ensure that a suitable room is available. Announcing such news in the middle of the ward is disastrous.

3 Ask the parents if they have noticed anything unusual about the baby.

4 Tell them the diagnosis by name (accompanied by suitable express-ions of sorrow and concern). Ask if they understand the term; they often have quite erroneous ideas, such as the child being a 'vegetable' or a 'spastic'.

5 Outline the prognosis for such infants, emphasizing that in infancy and early childhood there will be some differences from normal but they are not all that great and that the baby will walk, talk, be happy or naughty. The real problem is that of mental retardation. Stress that they will not be left alone to cope and that plenty of help is available. Then leave the parents alone for a while and return to answer questions.

6 Several leaflets are available for parents about Down's syndrome, but in arranging follow-up and support it can be difficult to steer a course between providing too much information too soon and not giving enough. Try to move at the parents' own pace, leaving the details until they are asked for.

Further reading

Drosar, D., Baskieuricz, A., Irvin, N., Kennell, J.H. & Klaus, M.H. (1975), The adaption of parents to the birth of an infant with a congenital malformation: a hypothetical model. *Pediatrics* **56**, 710.

Section II

Chapter 5
Physiology of the Newborn

Respiration

Fetal breathing

In humans, fetal breathing movements may be detected *in utero* by the 11th week of gestation. The breathing is irregular up to 20 weeks gestation, after which it becomes increasingly regular, and is almost entirely regular by 36 weeks. The human fetus breathes $30-70$ times/minute, and breathing is usually present for $30-40\%$ of the time. There is a rhythm of fetal breathing, with more breathing in the late evening and in the early morning. The percentage of each day spent breathing decreases considerably before the onset of spontaneous labour.

A fall in fetal P_aO_2 abolishes fetal breathing, whereas raising the fetal P_aCO_2 doubles the time spent in breathing; fetal asphyxia abolishes regular respiration and induces gasping. Alterations in the fetal environment may decrease or stop fetal breathing. These include bimanual examination of the uterus, hypoglycaemia, fetal infection and cigarette smoke; hyperglycaemia stimulates breathing. Pethidine and barbiturates depress breathing, catecholamines stimulate it.

Fetal lung liquid

Fetal lung liquid is not inhaled amniotic fluid, and has a completely different composition (Table 5.1). However, it is continuously added to the amniotic fluid, in near-term fetal lambs at the rate of 150 ml/day.

In the human, lung liquid first appears in the second trimester, but large amounts are not produced until the last trimester. The volume of lung liquid is $30-35$ ml/kg which is similar to the functional residual capacity (FRC) of the air-filled neonatal lung.

Onset of respiration

The first breath

Once the umbilical cord is clamped, the newborn is expected to establish and sustain a pattern of regular respiration within 60 seconds. Various factors are involved:

1 Physical stimuli. Individually, and in combination, these can initiate respiration. They include the influence of gravity, light, lowering the skin temperature by a draught of cold air, and simple physical stimuli such as flicking the baby's feet (p.115).

2 Chemoreceptors. The most important single stimulus in initiating respiration is clamping the cord, and the asphyxial changes which ensue. How this is mediated remains speculative, since in experimental animals respiration will start with the peripheral chemoreceptors denervated, although the brainstem centres are probably functional. After birth, however, the chemoreceptors do become sensitive to small changes in arterial blood gas tensions, and are of considerable importance in the postnatal control of respiration.

There is, therefore, no single event that initiates the onset of respiration, nor one single, controlling mechanism. The enormous sensory input at birth, the change in chemoreceptor sensitivity, the asphyxia from cord clamping, and an increased activity of the CNS all combine to make the newborn gasp and aerate his lungs. Indeed it is unlikely that for such an important function as the onset of breathing, only one mechanism would be involved.

Lung aeration

The normal infant breathes vigorously within seconds of delivery. He can generate inspiratory pressures in excess of 90 cmH_2O, but usually lung expansion takes place with a much smaller inspiratory effort averaging 50 cmH_2O Radiologically the lungs usually become aerated with the first breath.

Table 5.1.   Composition of fetal plasma, lung liquid and liquor amnii (sheep).

	Plasma	Lung liquid	Liquor amnii
Na^+ mmol/l	150	150	113
Ca^{++} mmol/l	3.3 (0.62)*	0.8 (0.2)	1.6
K^+ mmol/l	4.8	6.4	7.6
Cl^- mmol/l	107	157	87
HCO_3^- mmol/l	24	2.8	19
Osmolality mOsmol/kgH$_2$O	291	294	265
H^+ nmol/l (pH)	46 (7.34)	540 (6.27)	95 (7.02)
Protein g/100 ml	4.09	0.03	0.10
Glucose mg/ml (mmol/l)	152 (8.4)	113 (6.2)	304 (16.8)

*Figures in brackets are ionized calcium.

Clearing of lung liquid

The majority of this fluid is removed in the pulmonary lymphatics and capillaries, although up to 35 ml of fluid may drain from the mouth of a term infant during vaginal delivery. About one-third of the lung liquid left after delivery is removed by the lymphatics, and the rest by the lung capillaries which open up with lung expansion. The absorption is very rapid, since a normal FRC is established within 60 minutes.

Pulmonary perfusion

All the factors resulting from the onset of respiration, ventilation itself, the fall in P_aCO_2 and the rise in P_aO_2 will increase pulmonary blood flow, and each has an independent effect to increase pulmonary perfusion (Fig. 5.1). The release of prostacyclin (PGI$_2$), a very powerful pulmonary vasodilator, also occurs at this time, and almost certainly is of physiological importance in opening up the pulmonary circulation after birth.

Mechanics of respiration

The normal fullterm infant breathes at a rate of 35–40 breaths/minute. Taking into account various physical factors in the neonatal lung, this corresponds to the rate of respiration at which the calculated

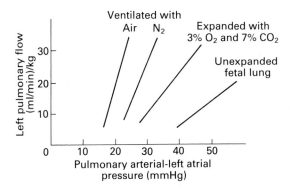

Fig. 5.1. Effect of expansion of lung with 3% oxygen and 7% carbon dioxide in nitrogen (equivalent to ventilation without change in blood gases); ventilation with nitrogen (equivalent to blowing off CO_2) and ventilation with air on pulmonary vascular resistance in mature fetal lambs. (From Dawes, 1966.)

work of breathing is minimal. Nevertheless many healthy surviving infants weighing less than 1.5 kg have respiratory rates of 50–60/minute for the first 2 months of life. The standard measurements of lung mechanics in the neonate are given in Table 5.2.

Control of respiration

Oxygen chemosensitivity

In a warm hypoxic environment (10–12% oxygen) an infant will hyperventilate for 1–2 minutes. After this, he hypoventilates and may even develop periodic breathing (Fig. 5.2). Periodic breathing during hypoxia is more common in premature infants, and may be seen in such infants breathing room air or even higher oxygen concentrations (p.162). Periodic breathing is not due to changes in $P_a\text{CO}_2$, since it persists if the $P_a\text{CO}_2$ is kept constant by adding CO_2 to the inspired gas mixture.

The reasons for this response to hypoxia are not understood, but by 5–7 days of age, hypoxia, as in the adult, causes a sustained increase in the minute and tidal volume.

Table 5.2.   Lung function in the newborn.

Measurement	Fullterm	Premature (if different)	Adult
Thoracic gas volume, TGV (ml/kg)	35–40	40–50	30
Functional residual capacity, FRC (ml/kg)	27–30	20–25	30
Vital capacity (ml/kg)	35–40		60
Tidal volume, V_T (ml/kg)	6–8		7
Alveolar volume, V_A (ml/kg)	3.8–5.8		4.8
Dead space, V_D (ml/kg)	2.0–2.5		2.2
Alveolar ventilation, $\dot{V}_A$ (ml/kg/min)	100–150		60
Minute ventilation, $\dot{V}_E$ (ml/kg/min)	200–260		90
Lung compliance, C_L (ml/cmH$_2$O)	5–6	0.5–3.0	200
Airways resistance, Raw (cmH$_2$O/sec)	25–30	60–80	1.6
Work of breathing (g/cm/min)	1500	500	16 000–50 000

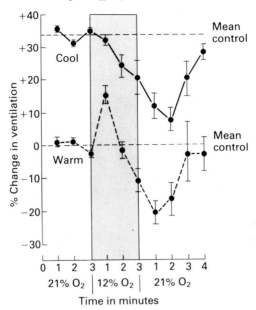

Fig. 5.2. Percentage changes in ventilation while breathing air and 12% oxygen in normal fullterm infants in cool and warm temperatures. (From Ceruti, 1966.)

In a cool environment, no hyperventilation is seen on exposure to hypoxia, and respiratory depression is the result (Fig. 5.2).

Breathing 100% oxygen for 30−60 seconds causes a 10−15% decrease in respiration which, particularly in premature infants, may progress to apnoea. If exposure to high oxygen concentration is continued for several minutes, after the period of hypoventilation there is a period of hyperventilation. The mechanism for this is not understood. However, breathing pure oxygen for some time may cause atelectasis in underventilated areas when oxygen is absorbed from the alveoli and there is no nitrogen left to splint them open. This may induce apnoea, since at low FRC stretch receptors in the lung may not be stimulated; conversely, it could cause the hyperventilation seen, since atelectasis may also stimulate intrapulmonary receptors to increase the respiratory rate.

Carbon dioxide sensitivity

In both premature and full term infants the arterial P_aCO_2 is lower than in the adult. The reason for this is multifactorial. The mothers, and therefore the fetus are mildly hypocapnic due to the respiratory stimulation of progesterone. There is a metabolic acidaemia following labour which stimulates the chemoreceptors; there is comparative hypoxaemia and there is the effect of cooling, which was important in initiating respiration. At term the peripheral and central chemoreceptors are functional at the low P_aCO_2 and the CO_2 response curve is left-shifted compared with the adult (i.e. the increase in ventilation with increasing CO_2 begins at a lower P_aCO_2). Some premature infants however have a flattened CO_2 response curve (i.e. the increase in respiration for an increase in P_aCO_2 is less than normal), in particular when they are having apnoeic attacks.

Pulmonary reflexes

1 Head's paradoxical inflation reflex: when an inflating pressure is rapidly applied to the lung, the infant makes an extra inspiratory effort before exhaling. This reflex is abolished by vagotomy, and the receptor is presumably a stretch receptor within the lungs.
2 Hering–Breuer reflex: the inflation component of this reflex (inducing apnoea following inflation of the lung) is present in the newborn, and is evoked by a gradual rather than the rapid inflation which evokes Head's reflex. The premature infant inspires for a longer time against an obstruction than does a mature infant or an adult, suggesting that inflation of the lung is required to inhibit respiration.

Chest wall reflexes

There may be marked distortion of the chest wall during breathing in rapid eye movement (REM) sleep in premature infants due to the loss of resting muscle tone in this phase of sleep. The more marked this distortion, the greater the discharge from muscle spindles, the more phrenic nerve activity is inhibited, and the shorter the inspiratory time; the infant can even become apnoeic. Reducing the distortion during inspiration by applying continuous positive airways pressure (CPAP) (p.164) increases the inspiratory time, and this may be the mechanism whereby CPAP reduces the incidence of apnoeic attacks in LBW infants.

Surfactant

The lungs are lined with a layer of lipoprotein which keeps the pressure constant within the alveoli irrespective of their diameter.

Lipoproteins which lower surface tension are known as surfactants. They are synthesized in type II or granular pneumonocytes in the alveolar epithelium, and are stored in the lamellar bodies of these cells. Surfactant is released by fusion of the lamellar body membrane with the cell wall. Surfactant is chemically complex (Table 5.3); it is 85% lipid, and 10−15% protein. The major lipids of alveolar wash surfactant are phosphatidylcholine (lecithin) and phosphatidyglycerol. Phosphatidylcholine is primarily dipalmitoyl phosphatidylcholine (dipalmitoyl lecithin [DPL]) which comprises 50% of all human surfactant phospholipids. The major route of DPL synthesis is the choline incorporation pathway (Fig. 5.3). Most of the disubstituted lecithin initially formed has an unsaturated fatty acid in the 2 position which is converted in the cell to DPL by transacylation. All the enzymes involved in surfactant synthesis have been identified in the fetal lung from the time at which surfactant-containing vesicles appear in the type II pneumonocytes.

The enzymatic pathways for lecithin synthesis are sensitive to cold, hypoxia and acidaemia. Postnatal exposure to temperatures less than 35°C and pH less than 7.25 causes a rapid fall in the amount of surfactant detectable in pharyngeal aspirates, and a halving of the synthesis of surfactant in *in vitro* lung systems.

Surfactant and type II pneumonocytes appear in the human lung at about 20 weeks' gestation. The amount present increases slowly until a surge at about 30−34 weeks. Detection of this surge prenatally (see below) indicates pulmonary maturity, and means that the infant should not develop RDS (p.130) when delivered.

Prenatally, the amount of surfactant present in fetal lungs can be assessed by analysis of the liquor amnii, comparing the ratio of

Table 5.3. Percentage phospholipid composition (mean ± SEM). (After Morley 1986.)

Phospholipid	Babies with RDS	Babies mature	Adult bronchoscopy
Phosphatidylcholine	61.7	80.9	79.0
Sphingomyelin	11.0	2.0	3.7
Phosphatidylglycerol	0.9	3.7	12.4
Phosphatidylethanolamine	11.7	4.5	2.6
Phosphatidylinositol	4.9	—	—
Phosphatidylserine	5.3	—	—
Lyso-phosphatidylcholine	2.0	—	—

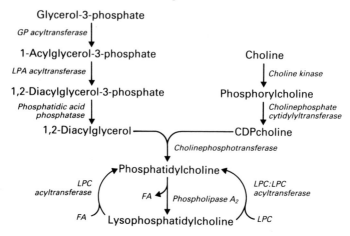

Fig. 5.3. Synthetic pathway for surfactant lecithin (phosphatidylcholine). (From Farrell, 1982.)

lecithin to sphingomyelin (LS ratio) and if this is greater than 2:1 the lungs are mature.

Surfactant synthesis is enhanced by steroids and thyroxine, and the fetal lungs in pregnancies complicated by intra-uterine growth retardation and prolonged rupture of the membranes mature more rapidly. Surfactant production can also be accelerated by drugs such as aminophylline and heroin.

At birth the surfactant has to be released and spread out on the alveolar surface. This is primarily dependent on ventilation and distention of the alveoli, but beta-adrenergic and cholinergic stimulation are also important. Surfactant, once released, has a half-life of a few hours only, and is removed by both physical and enzymatic means, including being washed up the bronchial tree in the normal fluid movement. The most important mechanism is probably its breakdown by lung phospholipases, the breakdown products being recycled as fresh surfactant. The rate of surfactant disappearance can be increased by breathing pure oxygen, and overventilation using inflation pressures above 40 cmH$_2$O.

Blood gases

In cord blood there is combined respiratory and metabolic acidosis. Within minutes of delivery the infant's $P_a\text{CO}_2$ falls to normal or below, and usually stays in the 4.25−4.8 kPa (32−36 mmHg) range for several days before rising towards 5.3 kPa (40 mmHg) by 2-3 weeks. The pH rapidly rises from cord values to 7.30-7.32, but then stays in the range 7.34-7.36 for 2-3 weeks before normal values of 7.38+ are recorded. There is also a mild metabolic acidaemia.

Table 5.4 gives average values for normal fullterm and premature infants for blood gases in the first month of life.

Oxygen transport

Fetal blood has greater oxygen affinity than adult blood, allowing it to become more saturated with oxygen at the capillary P_aO_2 values in the placenta. The position of the oxyhaemoglobin dissociation curve is controlled by pH, temperature, intracellular concentration of 2,3-diphosphoglycerate (2,3-DPG), and the variable interaction between these three factors and the haemoglobin present in the red cells. A decrease in pH and a rise in body temperature move the curve to the right, decreasing the oxygen affinity (more oxygen given up at the same P_aO_2). A rise in pH or a fall in body temperature has the reverse effect. An increase in 2,3-DPG decreases the oxygen affinity, and a decrease in the 2,3-DPG moves the curve to the left.

The position of the oxyhaemoglobin dissociation curve, and thereby a measurement of oxygen affinity of whole blood, is expressed as the P_{50}. This is the partial pressure of oxygen at which the haemoglobin molecule is 50% saturated with oxygen. For adult blood the P_{50} is 3.6 kPa (27 mmHg), and for fetal blood it is 2.6 kPa (19.5 mmHg). Normally, the fact that the infant's blood has a high affinity for oxygen (low P_{50}) is of little consequence. However, if the infant is unwell it is more difficult to assess hypoxia clinically, since cyanosis occurs at lower levels of P_aO_2 than in the adult. Fetal blood releases oxygen poorly, and tissue oxygenation may be sufficiently compromised in ill babies to justify exchange transfusion with adult blood to improve the oxygen unloading to the tissues.

Circulation

The fetal and adult circulation differ by virtue of the fact that in the fetal state there is a low pulmonary blood flow, a high placental blood flow and shunting of blood from the right side of the heart to the left side through the foramen ovale and ductus arteriosus. In the absence of lungs to oxygenate the blood, the fetal circulation is designed so that blood with the highest oxygen content gets to the left ventricle with minimum contamination by desaturated blood, and then passes

Table 5.4. 'Normal' blood gas values. (After Roberton 1986.)

	P_aO_2				P_aCO_2				H^+			
	kPa	mmHg	kPa	mmHg	mmHg	kPa	mmHg	kPa	nmol/l	pH	nmol/l	pH
15 minutes	11.6	87			28	3.7			48	7.32		
30 minutes	11.4	86			32	4.3			43	7.37		
60 minutes	10.8	81			31	4.1			40	7.40		
1–6 hours	*8.0–10.6*	*60–80*	*8.0–9.3*	*60–70*	36–45	4.7–6.0	*35–45*		46–49	7.31–7.34	*42–48*	*7.32–7.36*
6–24 hours	*9.3–10*	*70–75*	*8.0–9.3*	*60–70*	33–36	4.4–4.8	*27–40*	*3.6–5.3*	37–43	7.37–7.43	*35–45*	*7.36–7.45*
24–48 hours	*10.0–10.6*	*75–80*	*9.3–10*	*70–75*	33–34	4.4–4.5	*30–40*	*4.0–5.3*	42–44	7.36–7.38	*37–42*	*7.38–7.43*
48 hours–												
1 week	*9.3–11.3*	*70–85*	*10.0–10.6*	*75–80*	33–36	4.4–4.8	*32–36*	*4.3–4.5*	42–44	7.36–7.38	*40–48*	*7.32–7.40*
2 weeks					36–39	4.8–5.2			43	7.37		
3 weeks					40	5.3			42	7.38		
1 month					39	5.2			41	7.39		

The values at 15, 30 and 60 minutes are from unpublished observations on fullterm infants. Data from 1 hour to 1 week are drawn from literature on arterial samples, data beyond 1 week are based on capillary samples. Italic figures refer to premature infants; roman figures to fullterm infants.

to the coronaries and the developing brain. To achieve this the ductus venosus takes umbilical venous blood through the liver and a very short inferior vena cava with minimal admixture of desaturated gut blood. The superior margin of the foramen ovale lies over the entry of the inferior vena cava into the atria and directs most of the blood into the left atrium (Fig. 5.4).

The fetal pulmonary arteries are thick-walled and muscular, keeping pulmonary vascular resistance high and pulmonary artery pressure at, or slightly above, aortic pressure. This keeps the right ventricular

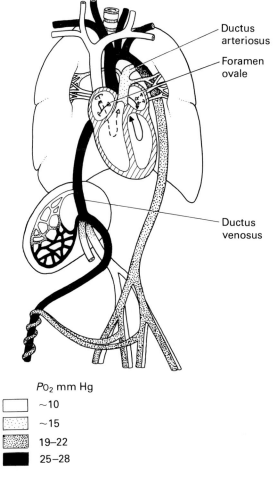

Po_2 mm Hg

☐	~10
▦	~15
▨	19–22
■	25–28

Fig. 5.4. Diagram of fetal circulation. Shading indicates the Po_2 of the blood. (From Rigby & Shinebourne, 1982.)

pressure high, and ensures that most of the right ventricular output bypasses the lungs via the ductus arteriosus.

Neonatal circulatory function

The fetal and neonatal heart rate is about 140/minute with a normal range of 120−160/minute. The blood volume of the term human newborn plus placenta is 105 ml/kg, and about 30% is in the placenta. Varying the time of umbilical cord clamping causes big variations in the infant's blood volume after birth with a range of 70−95 ml/kg. After late clamping the expanding pulmonary vasculature takes some of the volume, but the rest is taken up by vascular distention in capacitance vessels in the body and by cardiac dilatation. Some plasma water moves into the interstitial tissues within 30−60 minutes of delivery and is then excreted in the urine. By the second day, late-clamped infants still have a higher blood volume (93 ml/kg cf. 82 ml/kg) and a much higher PCV (60% cf. 44%).

Blood pressure rises steadily during gestation. At 28 weeks gestation the blood pressure is 45/30 and at full term 70/45. In the 2 hours after delivery the systemic pressure falls slightly. This is partially due to recovery from birth asphyxia, and partly due to the immediate postnatal circulatory adaptations to the placental transfusion. Blood pressure then gradually rises during infancy.

The distribution of cardiac output in fetal and neonatal animals has been studied in resting conditions and asphyxia. During fetal asphyxia the cardiac output falls and is distributed primarily to the placenta, brain and myocardium. The flow to these organs is sustained or even increased at the expense of virtually no blood flow to the lungs, gut, kidneys or muscle. In postnatal asphyxia the lung flow is sustained and there is no placental circulation, but otherwise the redistribution of cardiac output is similar.

Changes in the circulation at birth

Pulmonary vasculature

Throughout fetal life muscular pulmonary arteries remain vasoconstricted with a high resistance. With abundant arteriolar smooth muscle both *in utero* and immediately postnally, the pulmonary vasculature is very labile. With the onset of respiration, pulmonary ventilation, a fall in $P_a CO_2$ and a rise in $P_a O_2$, and increasing plasma levels of prostacyclin, each have an independent effect in causing pulmonary vasodilation (Fig. 5.1). The pulmonary vascular resistance therefore falls rapidly in the first few days.

However, in some newborn infants this does not happen, producing the condition of persistent pulmonary hypertension of the newborn (p.200). In others, hypoxia and acidaemia secondary to lung disease cause pulmonary arterial spasm, pulmonary hypertension and a tendency for the circulation to revert to the fetal pattern with large right-to-left shunts through the ductus arteriousus and patent foramen ovale.

After the initial fall in the first few days, the pulmonary blood pressure falls more slowly over the next month as the pulmonary musculature involutes. At 1 month the pulmonary artery pressure is only slightly higher than normal adult levels, and by 6 months it averages 25/5 mmHg.

Ductus venosus

The ductus venosus probably closes simply as a result of the reduction in blood flow after the umbilical cord is clamped. Angiography shows that it closes within a few hours of birth and it is difficult to pass a catheter through it more than 12 hours postnatally. Anatomic obliteration occurs by 2 months of age.

Foramen ovale

The right atrial pressure falls immediately after birth with the cessation of umbilical flow. Simultaneously the pressure in the left atrium rises with the increase in pulmonary blood flow following ventilation. These two changes tend to hold the foramen ovale shut, though in the first few hours and days of life, the pressure difference between the atria is only 2−3 mmHg. The foramen ovale remains potentially patent in 30% of normal adults.

Ductus arteriosus

The muscle in the ductus wall constricts when P_aO_2 rises. Oxygen is not the only important factor; prostaglandin E, hypocalcaemia, and a high pulmonary artery pressure all tend to keep the ductus patent, whereas adrenalin and noradrenalin constrict it. In both animals and humans the premature ductus is less sensitive to these factors and in particular it is much less sensitive to the effects of P_aO_2.

Constriction starts within 15–30 minutes of delivery, but partial patency persists for some hours or days. By the end of the first postnatal day there is intimal proliferation and gradual obliteration of the channel with complete closure by 2–3 weeks.

Temperature control

Physiology

The newborn baby loses heat by conduction, convection, evaporation and radiation. The neonate has a large surface area for a small body mass, and the smaller he is the greater the loss, particularly if he is naked.

Conductive losses are small since it is unusual for an infant to be laid on a cold surface. Evaporative heat loss is considerable at birth when the neonate is covered with liquor amnii and is in a chilly labour ward. Evaporation of the liquor, plus the other heat losses in a labour ward can cool the infant down by 0.5°F (0.28°C)/minute. Thereafter, evaporative heat losses may enlarge if the infant is in very dry air, particularly in VLBW infants who may have a transepidermal water loss through their very porous skin of 100 ml/kg/day.

The infant radiates heat to surrounding surfaces. When the nearest surface is the incubator wall, the effective temperature can be calculated by deducting 1°C from the incubator temperature for every 7°C the room temperature is below incubator temperature. A single-walled incubator at 35°C in a 21°C room therefore has an effective temperature of about 33°C. This calculation also applies to windows in nurseries where infants aᵢ cot nursed. Radiant heat loss can be minimized by using double-glazed incubators, a small Perspex shield over the infant in the incubator, or by dressing the baby.

The other major route of heat loss is convection to air currents around the baby. Even within an incubator the air circulation may be considerable and small neonates may only sustain their body temperature if one end of the radiant heat shield is blocked off to stop the draught.

The neonate tries to conserve heat by peripheral vasoconstriction and also by curling up in a flexed posture to reduce his exposed surface. However, neonates maintain their body temperature when exposed to cold primarily by non-shivering thermogenesis (i.e. generation of heat in brown fat by the hydrolysis of triglycerides to free fatty acid and glycerol). These pathways are exothermic and liberate approximately 10.5 J/g (2.5 cal/g) of brown fat/minute, warming the blood passing through the tissue. During brown fat metabolism oxygen is consumed and, if the infant is hypoxic, his ability to keep warm if exposed to cold will be jeopardized. The metabolic response to cold stress is inhibited by drugs, intracranial haemorrhage, hypoglycaemia and brain malformation.

Since oxygen is consumed keeping an infant warm, the ideal thermal environment will be that in which the oxygen consumption is minimal. This is known as the neutral temperature range. Below it, oxygen consumption increases with brown fat metabolism, and if the infant is too hot and restless some oxygen is also required for muscle activity.

Incubator/cot care

By measuring oxygen consumption, the ideal environmental temperature for naked (i.e. incubator-nursed) and clothed newborn infants of different birthweights and postnatal ages has been worked out (Fig. 5.5). This shows the benefit of swaddling infants and highlights the fact that naked LBW infants can only keep their body temperature about 1°C above the incubator temperature.

Effects of hypothermia

Surfactant synthesis decreases and its efficiency as a surface-tension-lowering agent is impaired at body temperatures less than 35°C. The hypoxic neonate with RDS has no oxygen to spare for brown fat metabolism and is therefore particularly prone to hypothermia unless the incubator is kept hot (Fig. 5.5).

Effects of high temperature

The newborn can sweat and vasodilate. Efficient sweating develops at 36−37 weeks of gestation most noticeably on the head, chest and legs. Above this gestation, at a rectal temperature of 37°C evaporative water loss can increase threefold. Low birthweight infants, if exposed to a rising temperature or a consistently high temperature, may have an increased number of apnoeic attacks. Premature infants have an increased mortality at too high as well as too low an environmental temperature. The cause of this is not known. However, it emphasizes the importance of paying scrupulous attention to the thermal environment of the sick newborn infant.

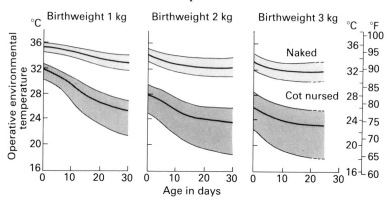

Fig. 5.5. Temperature at which to nurse newborn babies in a draught-free environment at 50% relative humidity. The dark line indicates the 'optimum' temperature and the shaded areas the *range* of temperature within which the baby can maintain a normal body temperature. (From Hey, 1971.)

References

Ceruti, E. (1966) Chemoreceptor reflexes in the newborn. Effect of cooling in response to hypoxia. *Journal of Pediatrics* **37**, 556−64.

Dawes, G.S. (1966) Pulmonary Circulation in the Fetus & Newborn. *British Medical Bulletin* **22**, 61−5.

Hey, E.N. (1971) The care of babies in incubators. In *Recent Advances in Paediatrics*, D. Gairdner & D. Hull (eds.), J. & A. Churchill, London pp.171−216.

Farrell, P.M. (1982) General features of phospholipid metabolism in developing lungs. In *Lung Development: Biological and Clinical Perspectives*, Vol. 1. P.M. Farrell (ed.), Academic Press, New York, London. pp.274−311.

Morley, C.J. (1986) The respiratory distress syndrome. In *Textbook of Neonatology*, N.R.C. Roberton (ed.), Churchill Livingstone, Edinburgh. pp. 274−311.

Rigby, M.L. & Shinebourne, E.A. (1982) Growth and Development of the cardiovascular system. Functional developments. In *Scientific Foundations of Paediatrics*, 2nd edn., J.A. Davis & Dobbing (eds.), William Heinemann, London, pp.373−89.

Roberton, N.R.C. (1986) *A Manual of Neonatal Intensive Care*, 2nd edn. Edward Arnold, London.

Further reading

Smith, C.A. & Nelson, N.M. (1976) *The Physiology of Newborn Infants*, 4th edn. Charles C. Thomas, Springfield, Illinois.

Section III

Chapter 6
Early Care of the Normal Baby

Care in the delivery room

Most births are spontaneous vertex deliveries at or near term, both mother and baby being cared for by an experienced midwife. With good modern antenatal and intrapartum care it should be possible to anticipate high risk situations which require a paediatric presence (see Chapter 14 for details). This section deals with routine procedures in the labour ward for healthy fullterm neonates (>37 weeks), but the same principles apply to all babies.

Resuscitation

Most infants quickly announce their arrival by breathing and crying within a minute or two, very little being needed in the way of routine resuscitation (see Chapter 14 for management of severe asphyxia). Fetal lung fluid is cleared after birth mainly via the lymphatics and capillaries, a small amount being squeezed out of the thorax during birth (p.29) The time-honoured practice of suctioning this fluid away is totally unnecessary for active babies who breathe within a few seconds of delivery. Virtually all infants are blue at birth but usually quickly become pink after a few breaths. If they fail to do so, oxygen can be given via a face mask, persistent cyanosis demands active resuscitation (Chapter 14).

The importance of warmth

Fetal metabolism produces heat so that the temperature of the fetus is about 1°C higher than that of the mother, the placenta functioning as a heat exchanger. Immediately after birth the infant is exposed to the relatively cold atmosphere of the labour ward and will inevitably start to lose heat by the means shown in Table 6.1. The most important factors are *evaporation* from the wet body surface and *radiation* to virtually every (cold) surface in the room. Drying the infant and wrapping him in a warm blanket immediately after delivery are essential to prevent a fall in body temperature. Details of temperature control and heat conservation are given in Chapter 5.

Table 6.1.   Causes and prevention of heat loss in the delivery room.

Heat loss	Reason	Counter measures
Evaporation	Baby wet	Dry with towel (preferably warmed)
Radiation	Many cold surfaces (e.g. windows)	Wrap in warm dry towel or blanket
Convection	Draughts	Close doors and windows
Conduction	Cold surface of trolley, cot or bed	Prewarm with overhead heater

Clamping the cord

During fetal life the placenta contains about one-third of the fetoplacental blood volume. After birth, factors which increase the volume of the placental transfusion to the baby are:
1 Delaying cord clamping until after the onset of breathing (i.e. lung expansion and pulmonary capillary filling).
2 Uterine contractions before placental separation, squeezing blood into the baby.
3 The effects of gravity with the placenta above the baby.
4 Delaying cord clamping for more than about 60 seconds.
    The timing of cord clamping is controversial, but in the healthy infant, not crucial. In most cases it seems logical to clamp the cord after the first breath or two and to avoid a large height difference between placenta and baby. Usually two clamps are placed on the baby end of the cord before cutting it (in case one slips off accidentally leading to rapid exsanguination). A plastic clamp is then applied about 1 cm from the base of the cord, and the redundant cord and clamp cut off.

Prevention of umbilical sepsis

The umbilical cord stump is a perfect culture medium for many ubiquitous bacteria and it is therefore common practice to spray the cord stump with an aerosol antibiotic spray such as Polybactrin, and to repeat this daily until the cord separates.

Vitamin K

The newborn infant cannot synthesize vitamin K in the gut until the bacterial flora are established and his intake, if breast fed, is very low. Clotting factors tend to be low and the infant is at risk from haemorrhagic disease (Chapter 25). Therefore it should be routine practice to give a prophylactic dose of 1 mg of phytomenadione (e.g. Konakion) to *all* infants at birth. This can be given i.m. or orally.

Blood samples

Do not forget to check whether cord blood samples are needed, e.g. if the mother is rhesus negative it is vital to know the infant's blood group. Blood is easily obtained from the placental veins and will thus save the baby from a painful prick later.

Examination

All babies should be checked soon after birth (usually by the midwife following an uncomplicated fullterm labour), but the paediatrician, if summoned to the delivery, should make a quick appraisal of the infant after any necessary resuscitation. This examination is generally confined to checking:

1 That the infant is pink and breathing well.
2 That there are no major abnormalities requiring immediate attention or explanation to the parents such as hare lip/cleft palate, spina bifida, anal atresia or ambiguous genitalia.

Babies are frequently smothered in blood and/or vernix making a detailed examination at this time difficult or impossible; undue exposure also leads to heat loss. For the same reason there is no need for a ritual bath at this stage. The parents may often be very anxious to know the baby's weight, which is perfectly reasonable; measuring the length, however, is wildly inaccurate.

Mother/family attachment: 'bonding'

This subject is discussed in detail elsewhere (Chapter 3) but never forget that the baby belongs to the parents and not to the doctors or midwives. It is a terrible reflection on our modern 'civilized' society that such basic instincts have had to be studied (with PhD theses galore) in order to establish the rights of mother and baby to be together. The denial of these rights has, in turn, led to the formation of vociferous pressure groups for home confinements, alternative 'birth centres' and the like. It is up to the medical and midwifery professions to provide a more individual and humanized atmosphere in the hospital. The baby should be given to the parents as soon as possible after birth so that they can kiss, cuddle and talk to him; no

attempt however should be made to force the baby on an unwilling
mother with the implied command, 'now get bonded'.

Care on a postnatal ward

'Rooming-in', that is keeping the baby in a cot by the mothers'
bedside for as much of the 24 hours as she desires, should be the rule.
She can then feed and change her own baby whenever he needs it and
respond to his signals and crying immediately — an important component of learning to care for him. It is particularly important to
recognize that breast-fed infants rarely have a 4-hourly feeding schedule, and that if the mother has her baby in his cot beside her, she can
breast-feed him 2–3-hourly if necessary (see Chapter 8).

The practice of herding newborn babies into nurseries for most of
the day and releasing them to their mothers for feeding and visitors is
archaic, inefficient and cruel. It compromises successful breast-feeding
and promotes nursery epidemics of infectious disease.

Chapter 7
Examination of the Newborn

Most parents expect their baby to be absolutely normal; they are entitled to be reassured on this point.

Purpose of the examination:

1 To check that the baby has adapted successfully to extra-uterine life.
2 To reassure the mother that she has a healthy, normal infant and to answer any question that she may have.
3 To exclude abnormalities that may need treatment at once or in the future.
4 To explain the nature of any such abnormalities or minor variations and to outline the probable management.

To interpret any neonatal examination you must have some understanding of the following general principles:
1 Possible effects of the intra-uterine environment (nutritional state, posture).
2 The influences of labour and of drugs given to the mother (birth trauma, CNS depression, etc.).
3 Physiological and biochemical changes during and after birth.
4 The immense number of normal variations and minor deviations encountered in the neonate.

Full routine examination

Always do this in the presence of the mother since a most important function is to answer her questions.

The following general format is recommended:
1 Check the maternal, obstetric and social history from the notes and from the nursing staff.
2 Always introduce yourself to the mother and explain what you are doing.
3 Examine the baby.
4 Give reassurance and advice.

Background knowledge

It is useful to have a mental checklist of relevant information before starting which should include:
• Birthweight and reputed GA, noting whether these are mutually compatible
• Mother's age, ethnic group, and social background
• Any chronic maternal disease and treatment?
• Any relevant family history?
• Outcome of previous pregnancies
• Any complications of this pregnancy?
• Any fetal distress?
• What drugs and/or anaesthesia were given?
• Mode of delivery
• Condition at birth; was any resuscitation needed?
• When did the baby breathe?
• Was he ever in the NNU, and if so why?

Introduction to the mother

Chatting to the mother before the examination serves several important functions:
1 Establishing a relationship between you, making the mother feel like an individual; asking the baby's name is always a good introduction.
2 Helping to gauge the level at which to pitch any discussion over problems.
3 Allowing observation of the mother's attitude to her baby.
4 Allowing you to observe the baby, noting his colour, breathing pattern, facies, posture and movements.

Formal examination

Undress the baby in a warm room or get the mother to do it for you. A 'system oriented' examination can seldom be performed. Take full advantage of quiet periods to feel the anterior fontanelle, auscultate the heart and palpate the abdomen. The order for the examination is immaterial. Leave the hips until nearly the end because testing them often makes the baby cry; the same applies to measuring the head circumference.

Throughout the examination observe the baby's posture, muscle

tone, movements and reactions to stimuli so that there is little need for a formal examination of the CNS.
A suggested order is as follows:
- Feel the anterior fontanelle for size and tension
- Look at the facies for colour or any peculiarities
- Examine the scalp and skull
- Inspect the chest and auscultate the heart
- Inspect the abdomen and palpate it
- Examine eyes, ears, nose, mouth
- Examine neck (including clavicles), arms, hands, legs, feet
- Feel for femoral pulses
- Examine genitalia and anus
- Turn the baby prone and examine back and spine
- Return to supine and evaluate the CNS as indicated
- Examine the hips
- Measure the head circumference

Systematic review

Skin

The neonatal skin has many variations of normal which often lead to needless anxiety for both mother and staff; occasionally it provides the first clue to an underlying illness.

Colour

Healthy, warm babies are pink all over after the first few hours. Initially they may be covered in white, cheesy vernix (yellow or greenish yellow if the baby is post term or has passed meconium *in utero*). *Cyanosis* can be difficult to evaluate particularly if the baby is pale (anaemia or peripheral shutdown) or racially pigmented. *Acrocyanosis* (peripheral cyanosis of hands, feet and circumoral area) is common in the first 48 hours — after that it may be a non-specific sign of illness. Very plethoric infants (PCV >65%) can appear cyanosed without being distressed. Traumatic cyanosis or bruising of the presenting part, sometimes associated with localized petechiae may be seen. Always take central cyanosis seriously.

Mature infants appear paler than preterm ones because of their relatively thicker skin; generalized pallor may indicate anaemia or shock; capillary filling time should not exceed about 3 seconds if the skin is warm.

Jaundice (see Chapter 22)

Jaundice is frequently seen on routine examination, occurring at 2−4 days in about 30% of fullterm infants. Pay particular attention under the following circumstances:

1 Onset in the first 36 hours is always abnormal and should evoke the Pavlovian responses — what is the mother's ABO and Rh group? Are there any antibodies?

2 If the baby is unwell in any way (lethargic, not feeding, vomiting, unstable temperature).

3 Coloured infants, where clinical assessment is difficult.

Skin texture

Note whether skin is peeling (common in post-term infants), nice and firm (normal), or very loose (intra-uterine growth retardation or de-hydration). Oedema is uncommon in fullterm infants.

Skin rashes

These are very common; most are benign, however alarming they may appear. Flat lesions are described as macules (<1 cm), erythematous (blanche on pressure), petechial or ecchymotic (do not blanche on pressure). Raised lesions are papules or vesicles (<1 cm), or blisters (>1 cm). Some of the common rashes seen in perfectly healthy babies are described in Chapter 28.

Head and skull

Heads can be distorted to quite bizarre shapes for the first few days by:

1 Caput succedaneum (oedema from pressure over the presenting part).

2 Moulding of the skull bones.

Feel the anterior fontanelle for tension and size. It rarely measures more than 4 × 4 cm at its widest points though this is very variable; the posterior fontanelle is often open.

Examine the *sutures*, particularly the saggital, for undue separation (up to 1 cm is normal); overriding (a 'step-up' feeling from one side only) is common but ridging at the sutures may imply craniosynostosis.

Palpate the skull bones; areas of craniotabes (like pressing on a ping-pong ball) may be felt but are usually without significance. *Cephalhaematomata* (collections of blood between the periosteum and bone) are felt as a softish bump over the affected bone (usually parietal) and do not extend across suture lines. They may take 6 weeks or more to subside.

Inspect the *scalp* for any injury such as forceps marks or lacerations from fetal blood sampling, scalp electrodes or scalpels.

Measure the *occipito-frontal head circumference* (OFC) at its maximum — the normal range is 31–38 cm at term; excessive moulding can result in a spurious measurement. If the head is unduly small, consider dysmorphic syndromes, congenital infections or isolated microcephaly: if unduly large, consider hydrocephalus, particularly if birthweight is at or below average; a large head with widely-separated sutures needs urgent ultrasound evaluation.

Face

Occasionally the facial appearance is the first clue to an underlying syndrome (e.g. Down's syndrome); the bloated face seen in infants of poorly-controlled diabetics is also characteristic. Unusual features should prompt an extra-diligent search for other dysmorphic manifestations although they may well be familial and a look at the parents should confirm this. Inspect the mouth for size and symmetry; the asymmetry of a facial palsy is more apparent on crying.

Ears

Inspect the shape, size and position and feel the cartilage. Abnormally small, or large, floppy ears are characteristic of several syndromes. Low-set ears are those in which the top of the pinna falls below a line drawn from the outer canthus of the eye at right-angles to the face (Fig. 7.1). Note any pre-auricular pits, skin tags or accessory auricles.

Nose

Inspect the shape of the nose and the width of the bridge; the distance between the inner canthi is usually 1.3–2.6 cm. Flaring of the nostrils is abnormal and generally indicates some cardio-respiratory disorder. Snuffly noses are quite common and usually without significance provided the baby can breathe normally during feeding.

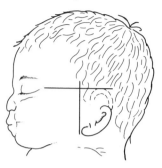

Fig. 7.1. In normal ears (dotted line) the top of the helix lies on a line drawn from the outer canthus of the eye at right angles to the facial profile. Low-set ears (solid line) are those in which the helix is set below the line. (From Gandy, 1986.)

Eyes

Inspect the eyes for any gross abnormality and check for any persistent strabismus or nystagmus. 'Sticky' eyes are very common in the first 2 days and seldom need more than simple saline irrigation; a purulent discharge needs bacterial investigation (p.173). Subconjunctival haemorrhages are common (analogous to skin petechiae). The sclerae provide a guide to jaundice, particularly in coloured infants. Examining the eyes can be quite difficult due to the strong orbicularis occulis; the best chance of seeing them is when they are spontaneously open, e.g. during sucking. The iris is normally blue or grey. Look for colobomata ('keyhole'-shaped pupil); if present look for other eye defects or dysmorphic manifestations. The cornea is normally 9–10 mm in diameter, a large cornea (>12 mm), particularly if hazy, may indicate congenital glaucoma (p.318). Look for cataracts. Routine fundoscopy is not indicated; isolated retinal haemorrhages may be seen and are not significant.

Mouth

Look inside the mouth either while the baby is crying or by making him open it (pressing down on the chin sometimes does the trick without protest). Avoid a tongue depressor if possible; ensure that the palate is intact. Minor variations of normal which may be seen include: Epstein's pearls (white blobs on palate or gums), teeth (which should be removed), short frenulum or tongue tie (which virtually never needs treatment) and rannulae (bluish swellings on the floor of the mouth) which are mucus retention cysts and need no treatment.

Neck

The infant has a relatively short neck; inspect it for shape and symmetry, palpate it for swellings, and test it's range of movements. Palpate the clavicles for fracture especially if there is any suggestion of an Erb's palsy, or following difficult deliveries (p.296).

Chest and cardio-respiratory system

It is difficult to separate the cardiovascular and respiratory systems because their postnatal adaptations are so inextricably intertwined. Start by inspecting the chest wall. Breast swelling is quite normal and not significant unless there is erythema; a few drops of 'witches milk' may be seen.

Many deductions about the cardio-respiratory state are made by simple inspection; colour is the single best clue to overall function. Observe the respiratory pattern. When quiet there should be no nasal flaring, no grunting, and no retractions; some babies, particularly if preterm may exhibit sternal or subcostal retractions on crying. Tachypnoea (rate >60 breaths/minute) may indicate pulmonary pathology but is also a most important sign of heart failure. All infants, especially premature ones, can have respiratory pauses of 5−10 seconds interspersed with periods of regular breathing. Auscultation of the lungs is an unrewarding exercise in the absence of respiratory distress. Palpate the praecordium for thrills or pronounced ventricular heave. Maximum cardiac impulse is usually in the fourth left intercostal space inside the mid-clavicular line. Percussion is not helpful. Check the peripheral pulses and always palpate the femoral ones. If these are absent or difficult to feel measure the blood pressure in the arms and legs to exclude coarctation (p.197).

Auscultation of the heart must be done when the baby is quiet; trying to listen to the heart of a crying baby is a waste of time. Count the heart rate, preferably over 30−60 seconds; after a little experience you will soon know whether the rate is abnormally fast (>160) or slow (<100). Listen to both heart sounds; the second is often loud and single shortly after birth, but splitting can be detected in 75% of infants by 48 hours. Note any murmurs, a transient grade 1−2/6 ejection systolic murmur is extremely common in the first 2 days without having any significance. Provided the infant is asymptomatic there is no need to mention it to the mother but it will need re-evaluation before discharge. Murmurs heard after 2 days need investigation (Chapter 17).

Abdomen

Inspect the umbilicus for discharge or peri-umbilical flare. The stump becomes dark and shrivelled and separates at about 10−14 days. Umbilical herniae are not uncommon but need no treatment and will resolve spontaneously. Look for distension and inquire about the passage of meconium; delay in passing it for longer than 48 hours after birth in a term baby requires careful assessment to exclude Hirschsprung's disease. Palpate the abdomen gently with warm hands when the infant is quiet and relaxed, if necessary by having him suck on a dummy or finger. Feel for the liver edge which can be up to 2 cm below the right costal margin in normal infants. With patience normal kidneys are palpable, but it is more important to exclude any abnormal renal masses or an enlarged bladder (Chapter 24). The spleen can often be 'tipped' but should not be more than about 1 cm enlarged. Auscultation of the abdomen is unnecessary unless gastro-intestinal pathology is suspected. Examine the groins for inguinal herniae (p.283).

Genitalia

Male

Inspect the penis for length (normal about 3 cm); occasionally it appears deceptively short, but palpation reveals a respectable organ buried in supra-pubic fat. Phimosis is normal and needs no treatment. Check the position of the urinary meatus, (see p.285 for hypospadias). Ask about the urinary stream; constant dribbling of urine is abnormal and may indicate urethral valves (p.284). Examine the scrotum and feel for the testes; at full term both should be palpable even if retractile.

Female

Inspect the vulva; the clitoris and labia minora are relatively prominent in preterm infants, but by full term they should be covered by the labia majora although the clitoris may still seem relatively large. White mucoid vaginal discharge is common and occasionally there is frank vaginal bleeding (oestrogen withdrawal).

Spine

Inspect the back for any obvious curvature and look for mid-line abnormalities over the spine or base of skull such as a swelling, dimple, hairy patch or naevus. Any of these may indicate underlying abnormality of the vertebral column or spinal cord (p.227). Mid-line dermal sinuses above S2 are rare but nearly always communicate with the theca and carry a risk of subsequent meningitis. Sacro-coccygeal pits, on the other hand, are common but harmless.

Limbs

Inspect them for shape, posture and symmetry. Babies who were vertex presentations usually have fully-flexed knees and hips but those who were extended breech presentations may keep their knees fully extended for a few days with the feet somewhere near the mouth. The tibiae are often laterally bowed and internally rotated. The feet and ankles may be in various positions usually related to intra-uterine moulding, especially if there was oligohydramnios. Polydactyly can be a familial trait, but look for other dysmorphic features. Digital remnants with a very narrow pedicle can be tied off with silk and left to separate by dry gangrene, but those with a broad pedicle should be removed surgically. Overriding toes are nearly always self-correcting and syndactyly is often familial; neither need treatment.

Observe spontaneous movements of the limbs; stroking them is sometimes necessary to elicit active movement. Move all the joints passively to test for their range of motion; due to intra-uterine restriction of space and activity the neonate may lack up to 30° of elbow and knee extension.

Hips

This is probably the single most important item in the newborn examination since early detection and treatment of congenital dislocation of the hip (CDH) may prevent long-term disability (Chapter 26).

Tests for CDH

These are quite hard to describe and are best taught by demonstration (Fig. 7.2). Have the infant lying supine on a flat, firm surface with the legs relaxed. Pacify him if necessary by dummy or finger sucking.

1 Straighten out the legs and look for any obvious inequality in length (in fact this is very rarely a feature of CDH in the neonate).
2 *Ortolani's test.* Fully flex the knees and flex the hips to a right angle. Place the middle fingers of each hand over the greater trochanters, thumbs over the inner aspects of the thighs and palms over the knees.

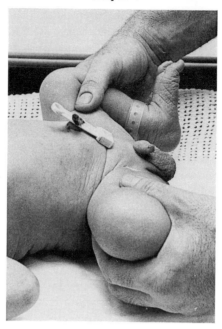

Fig. 7.2. Examination of the hips, see text for details. (From Gandy, 1986.)

Pull the leg away from the pelvis and slowly abduct and externally rotate the hips, simultaneously press forwards and medially with the middle fingers. A dislocated hip is indicated by feeling a 'clunk' as the femoral head slips forward into the acetabulum. When performing this test it is very common to feel (and even hear) a ligamentous 'click'. It takes a little experience to distinguish between clicks and clunks, the clue being whether there is any sensation of a jerking movement (clunk).

3 During this manoeuvre it should always be possible to fully abduct the hips so that the knees almost touch the couch; inability to do so may indicate a dislocated hip that cannot be reduced: presence or absence of full abduction should, therefore, always be noted.

4 *Barlow's test.* Hold the hips and knees as before. With the the hips held at about 70° abduction, test each hip in turn by pressing forwards and medially with the middle finger (over the trochanter), i.e. the same manoeuvre as the Ortolani test. Then perform the reverse procedure by pressing backward and laterally with the thumb (over the inner thigh), i.e. attempting to displace the femoral head out of the acetabulum. Normally no movement is felt, but a dislocatable hip will clunk out of the acetabulum and return there when the thumb pressure is released.

Following these tests it shoud be possible to classify the hip(s) into one of the following categories:

1 Stable with full abduction and no clicks or clunks = normal.
2 Stable with full abduction but with a ligamentous click = normal ('clicky hip'). Such clicks usually disappear over the first few weeks.
3 Unstable, the hip 'wobbles' about in the acetabulum on Barlow's test without actually coming out of the acetabulum.
4 Dislocatable, i.e. can be pushed in and out of the acetabulum.
5 Dislocated but reduced with a clunk on abduction.
6 Limited abduction on one side or the other or where abduction is less than 60° (possibly dislocated).
7 Dislocated and irreducible.

Notes

Category 2 can lead to confusion; if in any doubt repeat the examination in a few days or obtain another opinion. However, even when hips are meticulously screened in the neonatal period, some dislocations turn up subsequently (see p.294).

Central nervous system

Formal neurological assessment of the normal fullterm neonate is seldom needed, sufficient information usually being gleaned by talking to the mother and by watching, handling and listening to the baby throughout the examination. Some neurological responses vary widely according to 'behavioural state' (stages of sleep and wakefulness) categorized in the following stages:

1 Quiet sleep (non REM), eyes closed, regular respiration, no gross movements.
2 Rapid eye movement sleep, eyes closed (but making irregular roving movements), irregular respiration, frequent small movements.
3 Quiet wakefulness, eyes open, no gross movements.
4 Active wakefulness, eyes open, gross movements, no crying.
5 Crying, eyes open or closed.

Observations to be made during the routine examination (some of which are only valid when the infant is in an optimal 'state') are:

Posture (states 2 and 3). The undisturbed neonate lies predominantly in a flexed position; when prone the knees are often tucked under the abdomen. When supine with the head in the mid-line the limbs are roughly symmetrical. The fists are clenched and the thumbs furled intermittently.

Spontaneous motor activity (states 4 and 5). Normal infants move their limbs in an alternating fashion; they may appear quite jittery in state 5.

Vision (states 3 and 4). The eyes should lie in the mid-position and move conjugately; there should be no persistent deviation, strabismus or nystagmus. The infant can often be induced to follow a face (mother or examiner). It is worth telling the mother that her baby can see.

Hearing (states 2−4). The infant may startle to a sudden noise and will blink in response to clapped hands.

Cry. Pay particular attention if this is either high-pitched or very weak or excessive.

Sucking and swallowing. This should be obvious from the feeding history.

Muscle tone and power. This is tested by:
1 Assessing resistance to passive movements.
2 Pull-to-sit manoeuvre. Pull the baby up from supine by the wrists. In term infants there is some elbow flexion and the head comes up almost in line with the body (Fig. 7.3).
3 Ventral suspension. Hold the baby suspended with a hand under the chest. He should be able to hold his head in line with the body for a few seconds and to flex his limbs against gravity (Fig. 7.4).

Reflex responses. Numerous 'primitive' reflexes, e.g. Moro, stepping, walking and tonic neck reflexes as well as standard neurological reflexes can be elicited in the newborn infant, but there is no need to do them unless an abnormality is suspected.

Features which are rarely found on routine examination but which should arouse suspicion when present in infants with neurological illness and which merit more detailed examination and follow-up are:
• Persistent failure to suck
• Extreme irritability

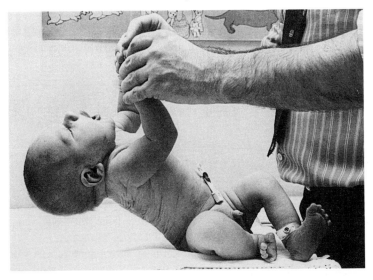

Fig. 7.3. Pull-to-sit manoeuvre. Note flexion of elbows and slight flexion of neck as the infant is pulled up by his wrists. (From Gandy, 1986.)

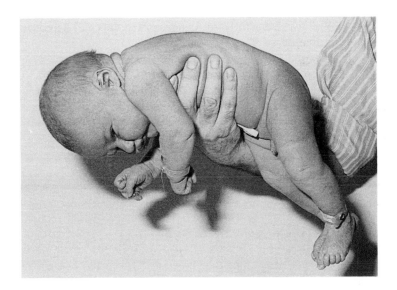

Fig. 7.4. Ventral suspension. Note the flexed arms and the head lying almost on a plane with the body. (From Gandy 1986.)

- 'Stary' eyed appearance
- High-pitched cry (often the nursing staff are the best judge of this)
- Abnormal posturing, e.g. opisthotonus, excessive fisting, obligate furled thumbs
- Generalized persistent hypertonia
- 'Frog leg' posture or generalized hypotonia
- Paucity or asymmetry of spontaneous movements
- History of frank convulsions or CNS disturbance after birth

Gestational age assessment

The cornerstone for assigning gestational age (GA) should be the mother's menstrual data combined with reliable early ultrasound estimation. Never rely on maturity estimated from ultrasound data that was obtained only during the second half of gestation.

There are many schemes for the clinical assessment of GA after birth, some of which purport to fix the maturity to within a week, but in fact they are only accurate to within ±2 weeks. Formal assessment of GA is unnecessary in the routine discharge examination of infants of 37 weeks or more reputed GA whose birthweight falls within the 10th and 90th centiles. Make an attempt to estimate the GA of LBW infants or others who seem inappropriately grown according to their obstetric data because:
1 They are at risk from different conditions to appropriately grown infants, e.g. hypoglycaemia in SFD infants.
2 The information is valuable in interpreting neurological behaviour and subsequent developmental progress.

The criteria used for evaluating GA after birth are based on:
1 maturation of certain physical characteristics;
2 maturation of the central nervous system.

Physical criteria

Some of the features which can be of value are given below (see also Table 7.1).

Eyelids. Remain fused until 25–26 weeks.

Skin. Dark red in very immature infants (<27 weeks) because it is thin and fragile with prominent blood vessels. It gradually thickens and by full term starts to desquamate with blood vessels no longer readily seen. Very fine lanugo hair is present initially and gradually vanishes by full term.

Table 7.1. Maturation of physical features in infants of varying gestational ages.

GA (weeks)	25	26	27	28	29	30	31	32	33	34	35	36	37	38	39	40	41	42
EYELIDS	fused		open															
SKIN:																		
texture		thin, gelationous		smooth			thicker									desquamates		
colour		dark red			pink							pale/pink				pale all over		
lanugo		all over						vanishes from face						shoulders		none		
plantar creases		none						1–2 anterior only					anterior two-thirds		to heel			
EARS: shape of pinna		flat							slight incurving				incurving upper two-thirds		whole pinna incurved			
cartilage		none							scant			thin			to edge of pinna			
recoil		none						slow				readily			immediately			
BREAST: tissue		impalpable											1–2 mm nodule			6–7 mm nodule		
nipple		barely visible									raised areola							
GENITALIA: male — scrotum		smooth			few rugae								anterior rugae			covered in rugae		
— testes				inguinal canal									upper scrotum			lower scrotum		
female	prominent clitoris, small labia majora												labia majora and clitoris covered					

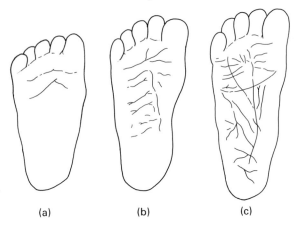

(a)   (b)   (c)

Fig. 7.5. Maturation of sole creases with increasing gestational age. Only of value if examined in the first few hours after birth: (a) 34–36 weeks, one or two anterior creases; (b) 37–38 weeks, creases over anterior two thirds of sole; (c) 40 weeks, creases extend to heel. (From Gandy, 1986.)

Nails. May reach the fingertips by 32 weeks and extend beyond them at term.

Plantar skin creases (Fig. 7.5). These can only be adequately evaluated in the first few hours after birth; they are absent in immature infants and start to appear at about 32 weeks. They gradually increase over the whole sole by full term.

Ears. Pinnae are flat with no cartilage in the immature infant and remain in bizarre shapes when folded. From about 33 weeks the pinna starts incurving at its upper margin; some cartilage is felt and the ear recoils after folding. By full term the ear is firm and fully shaped, with immediate recoil.

Breasts. These are non-existent in the very immature infant, with the nipple barely visible. A breast nodule with visible areola is palpable by about 36 weeks which gradually enlarges, and the areola becomes stippled.

Male genitalia. Testes descend to the inguinal canal by 29 weeks but are not fully descended until term; the scrotum becomes progressively more rugose.

Table 7.2. Physical criteria used in the assessment of gestational age. (Modified from Parkin *et al.*, 1976.)

SKIN COLOUR (estimated by inspection when the baby is quiet)	0	Dark red
	1	Uniformly pink
	2	Pale pink, variable over different parts of body
	3	Pale, nowhere really pink except ears, lips, palms and soles

SKIN TEXTURE (by inspection and by picking up a fold of abdominal skin between finger and thumb)	0	Very thin and smooth, gelatinous feel
	1	Thin and smooth
	2	Medium thickness, smooth, irritation rash and superficial peeling may be present
	3	Slight thickening, stiff feeling, cracking and peeling especially in hands and feet
	4	Thick and parchment-like, with superficial or deep cracking

EAR FIRMNESS (tested by palpation and folding of the upper pinna)	0	Pinna feels soft and easily folded into bizarre positions, does not spring back spontaneously
	1	Pinna feels soft along the edge and is easily folded but returns slowly to its correct position
	2	Cartilage felt to edge of pinna, though thin in places, pinna recoils readily after folding
	3	Pinna firm with definite cartilage extending peripherally, immediate recoil after folding

BREAST SIZE (measured by picking up breast tissue between finger and thumb)	0	No breast tissue palpable
	1	Nodule palpable on one or both sides neither being more than 0.5 cm in diameter
	2	Nodule palpable on both sides, one or both being 0.5–1 cm in diameter
	3	Nodule palpable on both sides, one or both being more than 1 cm in diameter

Female genitalia. Clitoris and labia minora prominent with relatively small, widely-separated labia majora. By full term, clitoris and labia minora are no longer so visible.

Some of these criteria have been quantified by scoring systems such as the Parkin score (Table 7.2; Fig. 7.6).

Neurological criteria

These are based on the development of the following four reflexes (Fig. 7.6):

1 Pupil reaction to light. This appears at 29–31 weeks and can be

66 Chapter 7

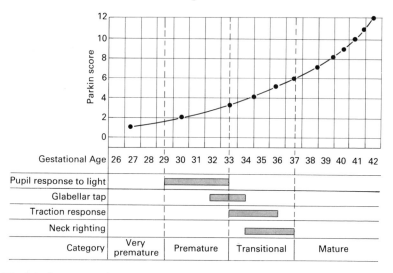

Fig. 7.6. Assessment of gestational age based on: (1) scoring four physical criteria (skin colour, skin texture, ear firmness and breast size) as described by Parkin *et al.*, (1976); (2) the appearance times of four neurological reflexes (Robinson, 1966). See text for details of definitions. (From Gandy, 1986.)

very difficult to see; the best method is to look through the magnifying lens of an otoscope head.

2 Glabellar tap. A blink in response to a finger tap on the glabella; appears at 32−34 weeks.

3 Traction response. Flexion of neck or arms when the infant is pulled by his wrists from the supine position; appears at 33−36 weeks.

4 Neck righting reflex. Trunk follows head when the neck is passively rotated in either direction from supine; appears at 34−37 weeks.

These physical and neurological criteria can be combined to estimate GA (Fig. 7.6).

References

Gandy, G.M. (1986) Examination of the newborn. In *Textbook of Neonatology*, N.R.C. Roberton (ed.), Churchill Livingstone, London and Edinburgh. pp.131−147.

Parkin, J.M., Hey, E.N. & Clowes, J.S. (1976) Rapid assessment of gestational age at birth. *Archives of Disease in Childhood*, **51**, 259−63.

Robinson, R.J. (1966) Assessment of gestational age of neurological examination. *Archives of Disease in Childhood*. **41**, 437−47.

Further reading

Dubowitz, L. & Dubowitz, V. (1981) The neurological assessment of the preterm and fullterm newborn infant. *(Clinics in Developmental Medicine*, No.79). Heinemann Medical Books, London.

O'Doherty, N. (1979) *Atlas of the Newborn*, MTP Press, Lancaster.

Scanlon, J.W., Nelson, T., Grylack, L.J. & Smith, Y.F. (1979) *A System of Newborn Physical Examination*, University Park Press, Baltimore.

Chapter 8
Infant Feeding

Introduction

Infant feeding practices have undergone rapid changes over the last century or so; from almost universal breast-feeding (even if from a 'wet nurse') the fashion changed in favour of the bottle, but there is now a welcome return to the breast and there can be little doubt that, for the fullterm normal infant, this must represent a 'best buy' in all senses. Nevertheless many millions of infants have been reared entirely satisfactorily on non-human milk (formula) although this needs careful modification to avoid some deleterious effects.

Feeding is such a basic need for the infant, and the maternal instinct for providing it is so great, that few things can engender more anxiety than symptoms connected with feeding whether it be refusal, slowness, crying, vomiting, or worries over the colour and consistency of stools. Early difficulties may well colour the mother's whole outlook on life and influence the relationship with her baby for many months or years.

Digestion

The neonate has to cope with a relatively large and dilute fluid intake to satisfy his energy and growth needs; *in utero* he swallows vast quantities of amniotic fluid and absorbs some of the protein from it. After birth his gastro-intestinal tract must adapt to absorbing all nutrients. Protein and carbohydrate are relatively well-absorbed, but most newborn infants have steatorrhoea and may lose up to 20% of their fat intake even if breast-fed. Artificially-fed infants have more severe steatorrhoea (up to 50% of intake), resulting in quite pronounced calcium loss in the stools. Marked steatorrhoea is also seen in preterm infants who have lower pancreatic lipase levels and bile salt production. Gut motility and sphincter control (cardiac and anal) are immature. It is hardly surprising that infants are prone to all sorts of symptoms related to the gastro-intestinal tract.

Composition of milks

There is good evidence that species-specific milk is tailor-made for its offspring in terms of nutritional, mineral and anti-infective components. Cow's milk has to be quite extensively modified to render it a suitable substitute for human breast milk.

Breast milk (Table 8.1)

Human breast milk is very far from being uniform and its composition varies greatly according to:

1 Whether the milk is actively expressed (EBM) or allowed to drip from the contralateral breast (DBM). DBM has a very much lower fat content than EBM and a correspondingly low calorie value.

2 Time of sampling during any particular feed. The 'hindmilk' has a higher fat content than the 'foremilk'.

3 Duration of lactation (postnatal age of the baby). The protein concentration tends to be lower in 'mature' milk than that obtained during the very early stages of lactation.

4 Gestational age of the baby. Protein concentration in milk obtained during early lactation from mothers of premature infants is higher than that from mothers of mature infants.

5 Maternal diet. The fatty acid pattern of breast milk reflects that of the maternal diet.

The figures given in Table 8.1 are for mature EBM.

Table 8.1. Nutritional and mineral composition of cow's milk, Cow & Gate Premium, Wyeth Goldcap Synthetic Milk Adapted (SMA), Osterfeed (Farleys Health Products), mature expressed breast milk (EBM), and 'Drip' breast milk (DBM).

	Whole cow's milk	Premium (Cow & Gate)	SMA Goldcap (Wyeth)	Osterfeed (Farleys)	Mature EBM	DBM
Cals/100 ml	67	68	65	68	65	54
Carbohydrate (g/dl)	4.7	7.2	7.2	7.0	7.4	7.1
Fat (g/dl)	3.9	3.8	3.6	3.8	4.0	2.2
Protein (g/dl)	3.4	1.5	1.5	1.4	1.1	1.3
Casein/lactalbumin	3.3/1	0.49/1	0.66/1	0.49/1	0.66/1	—
Sodium (mmol/l)	23	7.8	6.5	8.3	7.4	—
Calcium (mmol/l)	31	10	11	8	8	—
Phosphorus (mmol/l)	31	8.7	10.6	8.7	4.5	—
Iron (mg/dl)	0.15	0.65	1.27	0.96	0.08	—
Vitamin D (μg/dl)	0.02	1.1	1.1	1.0	0.01	—

Anti-infective properties

Fresh breast milk has many constituents which may help to prevent and combat infection including:

1 Viable cells, macrophages, lymphocytes and polymorphs — all excreted in quite large numbers.
2 Secretory IgA, particularly in colostrum.
3 Lysozyme.
4 Lactoferrin, an iron-binding protein which inhibits the growth of *Escherichia coli*.
5 Anti-viral substances such as interferon.

The stool of the breast-fed infant is more acidic than the artificially-fed one favouring the growth of non-pathogenic Lactobacillus bifidus rather than the potentially pathogenic *E. coli*. Most of these anti-infective properties are lost when EBM or DBM is pasteurized and/or frozen.

Cow's milk

In comparing cow's milk with human milk (mature EBM) the important points (see Table 8.1) to note are:

1 The calorie and fat contents are similar.
2 The carbohydrate (lactose) content is higher in human milk.
3 Cow's milk contains about three times as much protein as human milk and there is a marked contrast in the casein (curds) and lactalbumin (whey) ratio, cow's milk being about 3.3:1 versus 2:3 in human milk.
4 Breast milk usually contains more unsaturated fatty acids than cow's milk but the pattern reflects that of the maternal diet.
5 Cow's milk has much higher concentrations of sodium, calcium and phosphorus.

There are several dangers of using *unmodified* cow's milk or the older formulae (which are no longer commercially available) to feed neonates:

1 Hypocalcaemia; the high phosphate load leads to a compensatory decrease in serum calcium with a risk of fits.
2 Hypernatraemia due to high sodium content.
3 High blood urea and perhaps acidaemia due to the high protein content with a high casein/lactalbumin ratio, and the neonates' limited ability to excrete the hydrogen ions produced during protein metabolism.
4 Hyperosmolality secondary to the above, making the baby thirsty; this may then be misinterpreted as hunger so that more milk is given, leading to over-feeding and obesity.

Modified cow's milk formulae

The newer cow's milk-based formulae have been modified in the following ways to resemble mature human breast milk:
1 Their protein content and casein/lactalbumin rations are similar.
2 Their sodium, calcium and phosphorus concentrations are higher than in breast milk but not high enough to cause hypernatraemia, hyperphosphataemia and hypocalcaemia.
3 The butterfat of cow's milk is partially replaced by vegetable oils so that there are more unsaturated fats.
4 Iron and vitamin D are added.

In hospitals most infant formulae now come in liquid ready-to-feed form. For home use, however, powdered preparations are generally supplied. There are minor but insignificant differences in composition between the liquid and powdered forms. The nutritional composition of these modified milks make an entirely satisfactory substitute for breast milk in mature babies; indeed they may be preferable in terms of their iron and vitamin D content. See Chapters 13 and 20 for feeding premature and VLBW infants.

Breast versus bottle feeding

Although the aphorism 'breast is best' is often stated, there is actually very little evidence that bottle feeding is detrimental in the developed world.

In the developing world, where the risks of infant infections are high, breast-feeding is pretty well essential for survival. The anti-infective properties of breast milk are probably very important where mothers have major problems in sterilizing bottle milk due to:
1 The high prevalence of infection in the home and community.
2 The lack of an adequate water supply.
3 The lack of adequate equipment for preparation and sterilization of feeds.
4 Parental illiteracy thwarting their ability to read the instructions.
Furthermore, the family may lack the financial resources to buy the milk.

The other putative advantages of breast-feeding are as follows:
1 *Practical*. It needs no special equipment; the supply is always there, warm and convenient. Once successfully established it is quick, easy, efficient and satisfying to both mother and baby. Breast-feeding is cheaper than artificial feeding (cost of extra calories needed to produce the milk versus that of the formula, bottles and sterilizing equipment).
2 *Emotional/psychological*. These are somewhat intangible since many babies are bottle-fed successfully without undue evidence of emotional

deprivation. There is, however, no doubt that the increased body contact is satisfying to both and, since the infant often obtains most of the milk in the first few minutes of a feed, he spends a lot of time in non-nutritive sucking.

3 *Anti-allergic.* Cow's milk protein is well known to be antigenic and in susceptible families may lead to intolerance or allergy with diarrhoea, vomiting, abdominal pain and rectal bleeding. Breast-feeding may also reduce the incidence of infantile eczema and asthma in severely atopic families.

Breast feeding

Promotion

The earlier that propaganda for breast-feeding is introduced the more effective it will be, the aim being to establish it as the accepted norm in society, thus carrying it from one generation to the next.

Some influences on breast-feeding

Mother's own experience. If she has been breast-fed herself or has seen her siblings at the breast she is more likely to follow suit.

Education and propaganda. During the impressionable years of school these may have a favourable result. Mothers who have left school at 16 or under are less likely to breast-feed.

The influence of the media. This is now almost universal and could perhaps be further exploited.

Social mores. The attitudes of the husband, friends and relations towards infant feeding carry considerable weight. The overall increase in breast feeding over the past 15 years exhibits distinctive social class patterns, the incidence among class 1 and 2 is 80–90% whereas only 50–60% of class 4 and 5 mothers breast-feed their infants. Geographically the further south one goes in the UK the higher the incidence of breast-feeding.

Antenatal clinics. Overt propaganda at this stage is less effective than you might think, being more like preaching to the converted.

Postnatal wards. An occasional undecided mother may be nudged in the direction of breast-feeding by a positive and encouraging attitude among the nursing and medical staff or by sympathetic and successful mothers.

Physiology

The milk secreting apparatus (alveoli and lactiferous ducts) develops during pregnancy under the hormonal influences of oestrogen, progesterone and placental lactogen; some colostrum often leaks out during the second half of gestation. After birth, suckling stimulates release of:

1 *Prolactin* from the anterior pituitary which is the stimulus for milk secretion.

2 *Oxytocin* from the posterior pituitary which contracts myoepithelial cells round the alveoli thus releasing milk into the ducts. This milk flow mechanism is the draught, let-down, or milk ejection reflex and is vital to successful lactation; it has several other important features:

a It works most strongly at the beginning of a feed so that the baby may obtain a large volume in the first few minutes.

b After the initial flow the baby may pause in his feeding and then re-activate the mechanism to obtain more milk.

c The reflex is easily inhibited by fear or other unpleasant emotions.

d It readily becomes a conditioned reflex and the most appropriate stimulus for this should be the baby's cry.

e Oxytocin also contracts the uterus which may even be painful at the start of a feed.

The average British mother, once lactation is established, produces about 700–800 ml milk/24 hours.

Establishing lactation

Establishing breast-feeding takes time and patience and needs careful and consistent advice to maintain it. All too often the would-be instructors (doctors, midwives, health visitors) give confusing and conflicting advice on the practical management of breast-feeding; medical students are often taught all the theoretical advantages but may have little idea of how it is done in practice and even less on how to cope with the complexities. These problems can be mitigated by involving lay counsellors (e.g. National Childbirth Trust), or volunteer breast-feeding mothers in discussion groups of the interested parties and at parentcraft classes. It is also vital that similar continued support is available when the mother goes home.

Practicalities on the ward

1 Encourage contact between mother and baby soon after delivery since this is known to be an important factor (Chapter 6).
2 Avoid the unnatural practice of giving 'clear fluids' for the first feed.
3 *'Rooming in'*. The baby should be with his mother during her stay in the PNW. At her request he can be taken to the nursery, particularly, at night, to allow her some rest.
4 *Intervals between feeds.* The healthy term baby should be fed on demand with no arbitrary time intervals. Most babies will settle into a 3–4 hourly routine but if necessary they can be fed more often.
5 *Time at the breast.* There should be no clock watching over this. Never stipulate that the baby should feed for '5 minutes a side' then 10 minutes and so on. He should suck at both breasts for each feed but should start on alternate sides.
6 *Avoid test weighing.* Volumes of milk taken at different feeds vary enormously. Nearly all babies lose weight over the first few days (p.78) and there should be no anxiety-producing obsession over weight gain.
7 *Feeding at night.* Most breast-feeding mothers will want to be woken when the baby demands a feed at night. Do not give supplementary bottle or tube feeds unless she specifically requests it or the baby is at risk from hypoglycaemia (p.104). If the baby is howling and the mother declines to feed him he can be offered plain, sterile water, but see below.
8 *Stimulation of lactation.* The commonest cause of insufficient milk is lack of stimulus so if this is a problem the best solution is usually to feed more often, e.g. 2-hourly.

Getting fixed on the breast

The sucking action from a breast is different to that from a teat and the position of the baby is all important (Fig. 8.1). He should be held comfortably with his shoulders well-supported so that his chin touches the breast and his nose is left free for breathing. Pressure on the back of the head should not be used; it only makes the baby angry. It is not

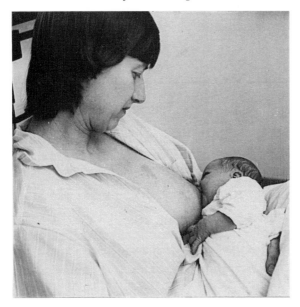

Fig. 8.1. Breast feeding.

necessary to get the whole areola into the mouth (some are much too large) but the jaws must be well behind the nipple.

Time and patience are needed to establish breast-feeding and the mother needs lots of help and reassurance if she is to persevere; by teaching her the principles she will gradually evolve her own technique. Experienced mothers will probably need little help, but first-time or anxious ones need plenty of support.

Some misconceptions about breast-feeding

Sterility. Contrary to popular belief breast milk is not sterile but contains organisms of the mother's skin flora; these are non-pathogenic.

Contraception. Breast-feeding is not a good contraceptive in the Western world although it may be a factor in the developing one.

Figure. Fears that the mothers figure will not return to it's pristine shape are unfounded, indeed she may lose weight faster after delivery if she breast-feeds.

Disadvantages and contra-indications to breast-feeding

There are very few disadvantages. Problems can arise in the first few days when relatively little milk is produced, particularly if the infant is at risk for hypoglycaemia (SFD, p.104).

The mother must always be present (unless she provides some expressed breast milk), The time and place may be inconvenient for exposing her breasts and the father cannot help with the feeding routine. The only absolute contra-indications are when the mother is taking the following drugs:

- Anti-neoplastic
- Tetracyclines (yellow staining of the teeth)
- Phenindione
- Lithium

Most drugs are excreted to a small extent in the milk but seldom in sufficient quantity to harm the baby. The ones most often called into question but which are safe are:

- Anti-epileptics
- Anti-depressants and psychotropics
- Antibiotics
- Corticosteroids
- Warfarin

Note particularly that warfarin is not excreted in breast milk and therefore it is perfectly safe to use it when breast-feeding (contrary to advice sometimes given from the older literature).

Occasionally, chronic maternal disease, e.g. very brittle diabetes, may preclude breast-feeding, although most such mothers can manage very well.

Breast-feeding problems

Engorgement

There is often some discomfort in the breasts when 'the milk comes in' on day 3–4. When the distension is frankly painful it is termed 'engorgement'. The condition is usually prevented by feeding on demand, i.e. keeping the breasts empty. Once established, the cure is to express the milk manually or by using a pump at the start of a feed. Demand or more frequent feeding then prevents a recurrence.

Sore nipples

These are generally due to the nipple not going far enough into the mouth so that the baby exerts strong suction on the nipple (like on a bottle teat) instead of having his jaws well behind it. The fault may be:

1 Flat nipples (poor prolactility). Prevention is by antenatal detection and correction (wearing of nipple shells antenatally).
2 Bad position of the baby at the breast.

If not corrected, the condition may progress to an excruciatingly painful fissure when the only treatment is to take the baby off the breast and express the milk until healing occurs.

Failure to fix on the breast

Maternal reasons. Flat nipples, engorged breasts, bad positioning. The management of these problems is that used in establishing lactation in the first place.

Infant reasons. Obstructed nostril(s), not hungry!, sleepy (e.g. sedated) ill, premature.

Insufficient breast milk

The most frequent cause in the early days is lack of stimulation:
● Not putting the baby to the breast early
● Only offering one breast at each feed
● Sticking to rigid intervals between feeds or arbitrary times on the breast
● Giving complementary bottle feeds

The mother may be tense, anxious, sedated, tired, in pain, or ill. She may be actually ambivalent about breast-feeding or doubt her ability to cope. Management is reassurance, support, patience, tact, understanding and giving consistent advice as well as attending to her physical needs. Putting the baby to the breast 2-hourly to stimulate prolactin production may help. Drugs to increase prolactin production (e.g. metoclopramide) are occasionally useful.

Duration of breast-feeding

In general, breast-feeding should last as long as both parties enjoy it. There is a progressive fall-off with increasing age but more women are continuing for long periods (Table 8.2).

Table 8.2.   Duration of breast feeding (% mothers).

	2 weeks	6 weeks	4 months	6 months
1975	70	45	25	18
1980	85	65	40	38

Bottle-feeding

Modified cow's milk formulae (e.g. Cow & Gate Premium, Synthetic Milk Adapted (SMA) Gold Cap, Osterfeed) are perfectly acceptable alternatives to breast-feeding in the developed world. In the developing world, however, artificial feeding may well be disastrous (p.71).

The brands on the market are all much the same; the one used depends on price, availability, personal preference or advertising techniques of the manufacturers. There is usually nothing to be gained by switching from one brand to another.

How much to give

The usual regime is to start with smaller amounts of about 20−50 ml/kg/day and increase this to 150−170 ml/kg/day by about 4−5 days; feeds are given 3−4 hourly. It is most important that the mother is given clear and adequate instructions about making up the feeds.

General feeding problems

Few things can engender more maternal anxiety than those connected in some way with feeding (see Table 8.3); the problems have to be handled with great tact and understanding and it is clearly important to avoid conflicting advice which serves only to confuse and perpetuate the problem. For breast feeding difficulties see p.76.

Normal weight changes

1 All babies tend to lose about 5−10% of their birthweight over the first few days and only regain it by about the tenth day.
2 After this, the normal weight gain for fullterm babies is about 30 g/day (200−250 g/week) for the first 6 months.

Wind

A small amount of air passes down the oesophagus with each swallow resulting in the formation of the gastric bubble; excess air comes up during 'winding' or 'burping' after feeds.

Possible reasons for excessive wind:

1 Crying before feeds.
2 Sucking in surplus air due to:
  a Poor apposition of lips to breast or bottle.
  b Bottle held in wrong position so that baby sucks in air as well as milk.
  c Hole in teat too small or too large.

The whole subject of 'wind' often assumes an inordinate importance in the mother's mind. So-called 'colic' is a frequent and mysterious symptom in which the baby, who is otherwise well, appears to have attacks of pain sometimes, but not always, in the evening; the condition is often attributed to 'wind' and is self limiting with time.

Vomiting

This is an almost universal symptom in babies but it is important to recognize the odd one who has significant underlying illness (symptomatic vomiting see p.251).

Feeble feeders (see also Table 8.3).

If babies refuse to feed or take a long time over it (>30 minutes), or consume far less than expected, consider the following causes:

Infection. e.g. thrush, upper respiratory tract infection, (particularly if the nose is blocked), systemic infection.

Systemic disease. e.g. renal failure, neurological problem, congenital heart disease (dyspnoea due to heart failure is particularly important and easy to miss if you do not think of it).

Abnormal (dysmorphic) baby.

Crying babies

It goes without saying that excessive crying is, at best, disruptive, annoying or worrying and at worst can drive the parents to distraction with the possibility of non-accidental injury (see also Table 8.3). Try to establish a cause and provide support for the parents.

Table 8.3. The table of F for feeding problems and fractious babies.

Feeding problems and failure to thrive	Fractious babies
Failure of lactation	Famished
Few feeds	Filthy
Flat nipples	Flooded
Fasting (maternal)	Flatulent
Fatigue	Feeble
Figure conscious	Frustrated
Faulty technique	Furious
Fanatical (class 1 and 2)	Febrile
Feckless	Freezing
Firstborn	
Festering	
Febrile	
Failure (e.g. cardiac, renal)	
Feeble	
Funny looking kid	
Faecal losses	

Stool problems

Physiological loose stools

There are enormous variations in the frequency, consistency and colour of stools. Transit time through the large bowel is relatively rapid and provided the infant is thriving there is seldom any need to worry, though reasurrance may be needed.

Pathological loose stools

Explosive watery stools may be accompanied by dehydration (loss of weight and poor skin turgor) or failure to thrive due to failure of normal absorption with loss of fluid, electrolytes and nutrients. Causes may include:

1 Infective. Gastro-enteritis is rare in the neonate but should be suspected if several infants on the same ward develop the squitters. Any systemic infection may lead to loose stools.

2 Lactose intolerance. Congenital alactasia is extremely rare but the acquired form secondary to almost any diarrhoeal state is relatively common.

3 Cow's milk protein intolerance (rare in the newborn).

4 Cystic fibrosis occasionally presents at this time with chronic diarrhoea and failure to thrive; the stools are bulky, offensive and fatty.

Failure to thrive

Failure to thrive in the neonatal period (Table 8.3), although common in the sick preterm infant, is a rare phenomenon in the fullterm one. There are four basic groups of reasons:
1 Inadequate intake:
 a Incorrect volumes being given or feeds not being correctly made up. For breast-fed babies see p.77.
 b Underlying chronic illness.
2 Abnormal losses from vomiting and/or diarrhoea (see p.252).
3 Underlying disorder, e.g. cystic fibrosis.
4 Abnormal baby (dysmorphic).

Diagnostic approach

1 Check weight gain against a centile chart.
2 Check type, amount, and making-up of feed.
3 Observe a feed. If breast-fed, particularly if the baby is several weeks old, it is justifiable to test-weigh in order to assess the milk supply.
4 Examine for underlying illness.

Further reading

Fomon, S.J. (1974) *Infant Nutrition*, 2nd edn. W.B. Saunders Co., Philadelphia.
Gunther, M. (1973) *Infant Feeding*, revised edn. Penguin Books, Harmondsworth.
Lucas, A. (1986) Feeding the fullterm infant. In *Textbook of Neonatology*, N.R.C. Roberton, (ed.), Churchill Livingstone, Edinburgh. pp.193–203.
Avery, G.B. & Fletcher, A.B. (1981) Nutrition. In *Neonatology; Pathophysiology and Management of the Newborn*, 2nd edn., G.B. Avery (ed.), J.B. Lippincott, Philadelphia. pp.1002–60.

Chapter 9
Prevention of Infection

It has been recognized for many years that the newborn infant, especially if born prematurely, is more susceptible to infection than older infants and children (p.170). For this reason, in NNUs in the 1930s–1950s, increasingly complex 'isolation' and 'barrier nursing' routines were introduced to minimize the introduction of infection and its subsequent nosocomial spread. With increasing knowledge of the organisms that infect neonates, and from whom they are acquired, it has now been realized that many of these precautions are unjustified.

Colonization of the newborn

Unless there has been prolonged rupture of the membranes or some other obstetric interference, the neonate is virtually germ-free at the moment of birth, but thereafter he is colonized with germs from his environment. That environment has two major components:
1 His mother; and most importantly the commensals or pathogens of her vagina and perineum.
2 The staff and equipment of the maternity hospital.

In general the mother is colonized by comparatively non-pathogenic antibiotic-sensitive organisms (and this also applies to fathers, siblings and other family members), whereas the staff are colonized with pathogenic, multiple antibiotic-resistant hospital-derived organisms. This is even more true if the infant is admitted to an NNU, which inevitably must be caring for the sickest and most infected patients in the maternity unit.

Contrary, therefore, to what might be implied from much hospital practice, the baby's parents and siblings are very much less of a microbiological hazard to him than are the medical and nursing staff.

Furthermore, it is crucial to appreciate that most of the practices aiming to minimize cross-infection in the neonatal period are designed to protect the healthy asymptomatic neonate from his apparently asymptomatic, but germ-encrusted attendants — the reverse of the aim in most hospital situations where cross-infection prevention techniques are being used. It is only when dealing with *infected* infants in an NNU that the infection control routines have the conventional aim of minimizing the dissemination of infection from a patient to staff and other patients.

Prevention of cross-infection in neonatal nurseries

Quite clearly, a basic standard of cleanliness and ventilation is an integral part of minimizing cross-infection in hospital, but the following general routines apply to the care of healthy babies in the PNW as well as to the intensive care of very sick infants.

Overcrowding

The more babies there are crammed into a given space, be it a PNW nursery or NNU, the more likely is infection to spread by some vector or another. Therefore admit as few babies to the NNU as possible (Chapter 11). Do not leave babies in PNW nurseries, but space them out in the ward with their mothers by encouraging 'rooming-in' (Chapter 6).

Mimimizing sources of infection

The following simple ward routines are essential components of reducing the risk of a newborn baby picking up an infection from his environment.

1 Keep medical and nursing staff with open infections such as boils or labial herpes away from newborn babies.

2 Encourage breast feeding: this not only provides the infant with many anti-infection factors (p.70), but also minimizes the small but constant hazard of nosocomial infection from the impedimenta of communal bottle feeding — though this latter hazard is largely eliminated by the pre-packed 'ready-to-feed' bottles of milk complete with disposable teats which are now provided by most manufacturers (Chapter 8).

3 Good umbilical stump care (p.46).

4 Isolate large, non-seriously ill neonates likely to be a cross-infection hazard, such as those with gonococcal ophthalmia, gastro-enteritis or superficial staphylococcal infections. The best way to do this is to put the baby and his mother together in a single room.

5 Avoid stagnant water, particularly in incubator humidifiers or resuscitation equipment, since this will become a rich source of *pseudomonas aeruginosa;* keep all equipment dry.

6 Do not use communal equipment, e.g. stethoscopes, blood pressure cuffs or thermometers, especially in the NNU.

7 Infants with septicaemia, meningitis, necrotizing enterocolitis or lung infection on an NNU are to some extent isolated from their environment by the incubator, and further isolation routines are not required. With such infants, however, hand-washing (see below) is of crucial importance.

Hand-washing

It cannot be emphasized too strongly that hand-washing transcends everything else described in this chapter as the single most important factor in reducing nosocomial infection in maternity hospitals and NNUs. If babies acquire infections from staff who are asymptomatic carriers of some organism, or who are the vectors of nosocomial spread from another patient, in the majority of instances, the infection is transmitted by hand.

Immediately before and after handling *any* newborn, a doctor, nurse or medical student must wash his or her hands using an antiseptic soap or an alcohol-based hand-rub. Similar standards of cleanliness should of course be encouraged in mothers when they are handling their own babies.

Before hand-washing, shirt or dress sleeves must be rolled up, and wrist watches and all hand-jewellery except wedding rings removed. Gowns, masks, and overshoes and the other paraphernalia of cross-infection routine are not necessary under normal nursery conditions, since they clearly have no effect on hand cleanliness, and long-sleeved gowns which are often used are as big a cross-infection hazard as shirt sleeves or dress cuffs.

If babies are being picked up and cuddled by people other than their mothers in addition to hand-washing the hospital staff should put on a separate gown for each baby to ensure that organisms on their clothes — either their own, or picked up from the baby — are not transmitted.

Parents and siblings who are well never need to use these protective garments, since they are highly unlikely to be carrying sinister pathogens — and if they are, the baby will in any case be exposed to them as soon as he goes home. Parents should, however, wash their hands before touching their own baby, and for obvious reasons must be discouraged from going around and handling other peoples' babies. Infectious diseases in the parents such as colds or gastro-enteritis may preclude or restrict their access to their baby, particularly if he is already sick or premature. Each such episode merits individual evaluation. In most cases, however, full contact between the mother and her baby is feasible so long as infected lesions are covered, a mask is worn to prevent droplets of a respiratory tract infection from spreading, and attention to hand-washing is even more scrupulous than usual (Table 9.1).

Table 9.1. Effect of perinatal maternal infections. (From Roberton, 1986, with permission.)

Illness in mother	Access to normal baby	Treatment
Varicella	Access restricted until lesions crusted; mother gowned, masked and gloved	Give 0.5 ml/kg ZIG to infant if maternal disease <5 days predelivery; consider prophylaxis with acyclovir
Zoster	Access	None: baby immune because of transplacental maternal IgG
Measles	Access	Give 0.25 ml/kg gammaglobulin to infant (hyperimmune if available)
Mumps	Access	Nil
Rubella	Access	No problem to neonate but keep mother away from antenatal patients and female staff
Herpes simplex (labial)	Access, but mother to wear face mask and treat lesion with acyclovir	None for baby
Herpes simplex (genital overt)	Access but meticulous hand-washing and gloves	Acyclovir orally to mother
Infectious hepatitis A (current)	Access	2 ml of standard immune globulin to baby
Hepatitis B (current)	Access	0.5 ml of high titre hepatitis B immune globulin stat. Immunize baby with HBV vaccine stat, with booster at 1 and 6 months
Hepatitis B carrier (unless mother HbeAg positive, when treat as active hepatitis B)	Access	Nil
TB (open)	Access	INAH to infant. BCG at 6 months if infant PPD negative or give INAH resistant BCG at once
TB (closed on treatment or in the past)	Access	BCG to infant

Table 9.1. (continued).

Illness in mother	Access to normal baby	Treatment
Syphilis (active)	Access, meticulous hand-washing, gloves for 24 hours	Penicillin to infant and mother
Malaria (active)	Access	Test infant's blood for parasites especially if mother has falciparum malaria or if the infant develops symptoms. Treat congenital infection with chloroquine
Acute enteric infections (cholera, typhoid)	Nil during acute phase – mother too ill	Nil. Encourage breast feeding if possible. Immunize infant
Leprosy	Access	Continue maternal treatment
Other tropical diseases (i.e. trypanosomiasis, schistosomiasis filariasis)	Access	Nil, but consult local tropical diseases hospital if infant symptomatic
Chlamydia	Access	Nil
CMV	Access	Nil
Acute respiratory infection (RSV flu)	Access with masking and hand-washing	Nil
Streptococcal illness or carriage	Access. Mask for group A strep. respiratory infection, hand-washing for all	Nil

Chapter 10
Biochemical Screening Procedures in the Neonate

The current biochemical screening procedures routinely carried out on all newborn babies in the UK are those for phenylketonuria and hypothyroidism.

Phenylketonuria (incidence 1:10 000 approx.)

All babies at 6−9 days of age have a heel prick blood sample analysed for phenylalanine to exclude phenlyketonuria (PKU). Ideally, the infant should be taking feeds normally. If, at 6−9 days he is on an inadequate milk, and thus an inadequate protein intake, he should be retested when his milk intake is normal.

In the Guthrie bacterial inhibition assay, the first test described and still widely-used, the blood is collected onto an absorbent card (Fig. 10.1) and the amount of phenylalanine present is assayed by its ability to support the growth of Bacillus subtilis on an agar plate containing β-thienylalanine. This compound inhibits the growth of Bacillus subtilis unless its effect is counteracted by an increased phenylalanine level in the blood spot. Approximately 1 in 2000 of all infants are positive on screening. They are recalled, and their plasma phenylalanine remeasured to confirm whether they have classical PKU, one of the other forms of persistent hyperphenylalaninaemia, including 'malignant' PKU (a rare condition due to a co-factor deficiency) or simply transient hyperphenylalaninaemia associated with metabolic immaturity or a high protein intake.

If PKU or a variant is confirmed by a second high phenylalanine level the baby should be referred to a specialist centre for a full investigation and stabilization on diet.

Hypothyroidism (incidence 1:3500 approx.)

Screening for this condition is now routine in Britain. Using one of the blood spots collected at 6 days on the Guthrie card (Fig. 10.1) radioimmunoassay is done for thyroid-stimulating hormone (TSH) and/or thyroxine (T_4). When a primary T_4 test is used, infants whose level falls in the lower 10−20% of values (varying with local practice)

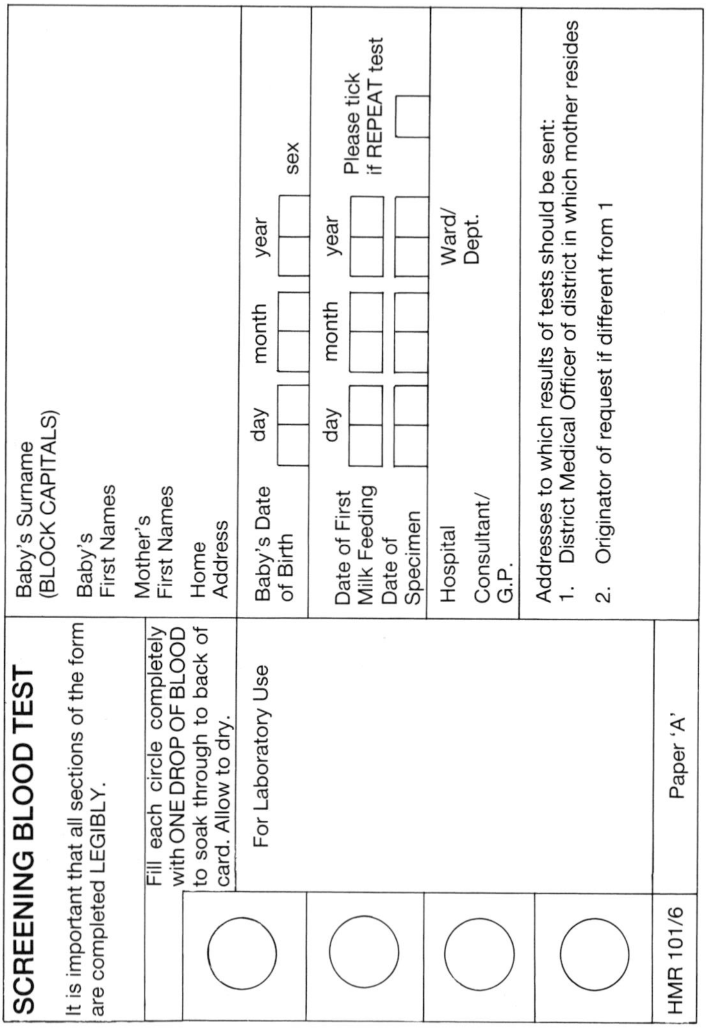

Fig. 10.1. Card currently used for collection of blood for Guthrie Tests.

have another of the spots analysed for TSH, also by radioimmunoassay. Those with a low T_4 and high TSH are then recalled for further evaluation. This is required in about 0.2–0.3% of all infants tested. The incidence of hypothyroidism detected in this way is about double that previously identified in retrospective surveys, presumably due to the fact that some neonates, particularly if preterm, have transient hypothyroidism, whereas others have only marginally subnormal thyroid function which would otherwise not have become clinically apparent until later in childhood. All infants confirmed as hypothyroid should be treated (p.274), and carefully followed up.

Other aminoacidopathies

In some parts of the UK, and elsewhere in the world, other aminoacidopathies such as maple syrup urine disease, homocystinuria, histidinaemia and tyrosinaemia are screened for, either by modifications of the Guthrie bacterial inhibition type of assay, or by plasma chromatography or fluorimetry.

However, these conditions (Table 10.1) are all rare, difficult to treat, or, in the case of histidinaemia, of doubtful clinical significance. It is questionable therefore, whether the addition of extra screening tests for these conditions is cost-effective.

Galactosaemia (incidence 1:40–60 000)

Infants with this condition may become ill in the neonatal period before screening can be carried out. However, the test for galactose-1-phosphate uridyl transferase deficiency is easily and cheaply carried

Table 10.1.   Rare aminoacidopathies.

Condition	Incidence	Reason for not screening
Histidinaemia	1:17 000	Treatment unneccessary
Homocystinuria	1:150 000	Rare: doubtful if presymptomatic treatment is beneficial
Maple syrup urine disease	1:250 000	Rare. Even early dietary treatment leaves most patients severely handicapped
Tyrosinaemia	Very rare except in Quebec and Scandinavia	Too rare to be justified in Britain

out on red cells from a Guthrie or other blood specimen, and despite
the comparative rarity of galactosaemia it is probably worth while to
carry out routine population screening.

Cystic fibrosis (incidence 1:2000)

This is the commonest lethal inherited disease in Britain. Whether or
not neonatal screening is justified hinges largely on whether there are
benefits from detecting and treating this condition in its pre-
symptomatic stage. Opinions are divided at the moment. Originally,
screening was carried out by testing for albumin in the first specimen
of meconium passed by the neonate. This test was inaccurate, and has
now been replaced by a blood test. Most neonates with cystic fibrosis
have markedly raised plasma trypsin levels, and one of the blood spots
obtained at 6 days from the Guthrie test (Fig. 10.1) can be analysed
for immunoreactive trypsin (IRT). Preliminary studies suggest that
the test is specific with a recall rate of only 0.5%, and very few false
positive or negative results.

Section IV

Chapter 11
Admission and Discharge Policies
for Neonatal Units

A mother has waited 9 months to have her newborn baby with her; he should not be taken from her unless there is an overwhelming reason for doing so. Every maternity unit should ensure, therefore, that only those neonates for whom it is genuinely necessary are admitted to the NNU, and, of course, at the same time provide the family with maximum access to their baby (Chapter 3). Once a baby on the NNU is well, every effort should be made to discharge him home or to his mother on the PNW.

There are only three reasons for separating a mother and her newborn baby:

1 Severe maternal illness which makes her incapable of caring for her baby — though in most cases the normal term baby can be cared for by the midwives on the mother's ward so that she can see him as much as possible.

2 Illness in a baby which cannot be coped with on a PNW.

3 A birthweight less than 1.6–1.8 kg. Such babies usually need the warmer environment of an NNU, and often need special feeding regimes such as 1–2-hourly feeds, often by tube.

Avoiding NNU admission (Table 11.1)

Babies >2.5 kg birthweight

Too many of these babies are unnecessarily admitted to an NNU and separated from their mothers. Only about 2% of babies of this birthweight need NNU care; in particular there is no routine need to admit infants who:

1 Were delivered by caesarean section, forceps or the breech, or in any other abnormal way so long as they are in good condition after delivery.

2 Required a short (less than 5–10 minutes) period of IPPV for resuscitation at birth, but are normal by 10 minutes of age.

3 Have diabetic mothers (p.270).

4 Have congenital malformations which are not going to be life-threatening, e.g. Down's syndrome, hare lip, limb defects.

93

5 Have mothers with various long-term illnesses such as epilepsy, asthma, ulcerative colitis or heart disease — but who nevertheless produce normal babies.

In addition the majority of infants who develop the following minor complications in the neonatal period can normally be kept with their mothers on a PNW:

- Jaundice, including the use of phototherapy (p.257)
- Sticky eye/conjunctivitis (p.173)
- Thrush and other minor superficial skin sepsis (p.172)
- Feeding problems (p.78)

Babies 1.8—2.5 kg

Infants of this birthweight who are asymptomatic immediately after delivery can be managed with their mothers on the PNW (Table 11.1). Many of these babies are SFD (p.98) and therefore at risk from hypoglycaemia (p.103). To make it safe for them on a PNW, the nurses must be able to carry out heel prick Dextrostix estimations (p.103).

The conditions which develop later in the neonatal period in larger infants (see above) and can be managed on the PNW, can also be managed on the PNW in infants of lower birthweight. In addition some LBW infants require tube feeds to prevent early hypoglycaemia, or while breast-feeding is established; this can also be done in the nursery of a PNW with great safety, often by the mother under supervision from the nursing staff.

Early discharge

Infants with transient neonatal illness

Some infants above 1.8 kg birthweight, including those who are fullterm, *do* require admission to an NNU but have an illness lasting a few days only. As well as maximizing mother–baby contact while these neonates are on the NNU (Chapter 3) they can and should be transferred out of the NNU to their mothers on the PNW as soon as possible. (Table 11.1) Alternatively if their mothers have gone home the babies, once asymptomatic, can follow suit.

Asymptomatic infants 1.8—2.5 kg

These infants, cared for on a PNW, can be discharged as soon as they

Table 11.1. Number of babies admitted to an NNU at different birthweights, Cambridge Maternity Hospital, 1980.

BW	Total live births	Never admitted to NNU	Transferred from NNU to PNW (age on transfer)	Always on NNU
1.5−1.99	79	5	31 (4.6 days)	43[*]
2.0−2.49	194	159	28 (3.6 days)	7
≥2.5	3879	3791	76 (2.7 days)	12

[*]Includes 21 transferred back to the hospital, which had referred the mother antenatally or the baby postnatally. These were transferred at an average age of 7 days and a weight of 1.59 kg.

are feeding satisfactorily, and have shown that they are capable of sustaining their body temperature in a room between 21−24°C (70−75°F). It is very nice to know that they are gaining weight, but particularly if babies at the upper end of this birthweight range are feeding well by 2−3 days of age, it can be assumed that they will gain weight, and it is safe for them to be discharged. The midwife and the GP who, between them, are responsible for the continuing care of the mother and baby in the early puerperium can then ensure that adequate feeding is sustained and the weight gain is normal.

Infants <1.8 kg birthweight

Much the same principles apply to babies of this birthweight. There is absolutely no need to be doctrinaire about such babies achieving a specific birthweight before they are discharged home from an NNU. Once they can nipple-feed satisfactorily, sustain their body temperatures at environmental room temperatures, and have shown over a period of days or weeks that they are gaining weight satisfactorily, particularly if this has been largely under the care and supervision of their mother in the neonatal unit, then it is perfectly safe to discharge them. In Europe, North America and Africa, infants weighing 1.5−1.6 kg have been discharged home very successfully. This considerably reduces their stay in hospital, the effects of prolonged mother−baby separation, and also the cost of neonatal care.

Chapter 12
The Low Birthweight Infant. Incidence, Aetiology and Obstetric Management

In Britain in the 1980s about 7% of all live-born infants weigh less than 2.5 kg at birth. About one-third of these are SFD, i.e. below the third centile of birthweight for their gestation; the remaining two-thirds are truly premature (Chapter 2).

Prematurity

Incidence

Of the 10% of all newborn infants who are less than 37 weeks gestation, 40–50% weigh more than 2.5 kg at birth, and 70–75% weigh more than 2.0 kg at birth. These larger preterm babies pose comparatively few problems in the neonatal period, and the majority can usually be cared for by their mothers on a PNW (Chapter 11). 2–2.5% of all infants weigh less than 2.0 kg at birth, and the lower the birthweight of such an infant the more likely he is to suffer from one of the neonatal illnessess described in Section V. About 70% of the infants who weigh less than 1.5 kg at birth (VLBW infants, Chapter 2) develop some form of respiratory illness, and it is in infants of this birthweight that most neonatal morbidity and mortality occurs.

Aetiology of prematurity

If prematurity could be eliminated, much neonatal morbidity and mortality could be avoided. As yet the disciplines of obstetrics, endocrinology and epidemiology have come up with little that offers hope of preventing premature delivery, primarily because the physiology of normal labour, never mind abnormal preterm labour, remains unresolved.

The major causes for preterm delivery are:
1 Deliberate intervention by the obstetrician in the interests of fetal or maternal health, for example:
a Severe rhesus disease.
b Severe maternal illness — malignant disease, heart disease, hypertension, renal disease, infection.

c Severe pre-eclampsia or eclampsia.

d Evidence of fetal compromise, e.g. abnormal fetal heart rate patterns, fetal growth retardation.

2 Antepartum haemorrhage — either from placental separation or placenta previa.

3 Uterine abnormalities, e.g. bicornuate uterus, or post-myomectomy.

4 Cervical incompetence.

5 Spontaneous onset of preterm labour with or without rupture of the membranes.

Spontaneous onset of preterm labour is much more common in women from poorer socio-economic backgrounds. Why this is so remains a mystery. Various factors such as poor general health, smoking, inadequate nutrition, genital infection, sexual habits, and the need to do hard, physical work during pregnancy have all been suggested, but there is increasing evidence to suggest that local infection is very important, both by damaging the fetal membranes and by stimulating the release of prostaglandins and thereby stimulating uterine contraction.

Obstetric management of premature infants

As the results of neonatal intensive care improve, and offer neurologically intact survival for the majority of VLBW babies (Chapter 31), it has become clear that a major determinant of whether or not a VLBW baby survives or is handicapped, is whether or not he suffers intrapartum asphyxia. There is an important extra implication of asphyxia at short gestation — the effect on surfactant, and thus on the incidence of RDS (p.130). Surfactant synthesis is pH-sensitive, and an asphyxiated preterm infant is, therefore, more likely to develop severe RDS and its sequelae including a periventricular haemorrhage, than a non-asphyxiated one.

At gestations of 28 weeks or more it is reasonable for a neonatologist to tell an obstetrician, 'give me a baby in good condition (i.e. not asphyxiated or traumatized), and I will give you a neurologically intact survivor'.

Conduct of labour

When an obstetrician takes the view that labour, late in the second trimester or early in the third trimester, is likely to produce a non-viable human being, then the neonatal outcome worsens both in terms of morbidity and mortality. Therefore in all labours likely to produce a viable infant at more than 26 weeks gestation, the obstetrician should apply the same standards of intrapartum care and monitoring, including fetal cardiotocography and fetal scalp blood sampling for pH, that he would in a term infant who was at risk. A senior obstetrician should be present at the delivery of all preterm infants. A wide episiotomy should be carried out to protect the frail preterm head, but forceps application with the same aim is not justified.

Breech delivery

At gestations less than 32 weeks the consensus view is that vaginal breech delivery is contra-indicated and such infants should therefore be delivered by caesarean section.

Caesarean section

Despite the fact that this operation is technically more demanding at short gestations when the lower segment of the uterus has not yet formed, the indications for caesarean section should be the same as at term, with the addition of routine caesarean section for all preterm breech presentations. A classical caesarean section may be justified in some instances. Furthermore at gestations above 26−28 weeks it is perfectly legitimate to remove the fetus by caesarean section from a woman with some complication — typically pre-eclampsia — when immediate termination of the pregnancy is necessary in the maternal interest.

It is doubtful if the oft-quoted increase in the incidence of RDS in infants delivered by caesarean section is true at short gestations, and this theoretical hazard should certainly not be cited as a contra-indication to the procedure in women less than 30−32 weeks pregnant.

Small for dates infants

Definition and diagnosis

The usual definition of an SFD infant is one who is below the third centile for weight for his gestation; by definition therefore, 3% of all newborn infants are SFD (an alternative [p.7] is to use below 2 SD from the mean, ≡ 2.3rd centile, in which case 2.3% of all neonates are SFD). Use centile charts which are derived from data obtained by measuring babies from appropriate socio-economic, geographical and ethnic populations. It is clearly nonsense to apply growth charts derived from a tall, well-fed sea-level population such as the Canadians to a short, light, high-altitude population such as the Nepalese. The weight of all newborn infants should be plotted on an appropriate chart as soon after delivery as possible, so that SFD infants are recognized and treated appropriately.

Four groups of SFD infants can be recognized:

1 Mature SFD infants lacking subcutaneous tissue who are wizened, wide-eyed and alert, but have a normal length and head-circumference. They suffered fetal malnutrition and reduced deposition of subcutaneous fat and glycogen late in gestation. Some infants with this appearance weigh more than the third centile for their gestation; these should be recognized clinically and treated as SFD babies.

2 Less obviously wasted, shorter SFD infants. They probably suffered more prolonged placental insufficiency which impaired linear growth more than fat deposition.

3 Twins and higher multiples.

4 2–3% of all SFD infants have a major malformation or some fetal illness such as Down's syndrome, congenital rubella, tracheo-oesophageal fistula, or congenital thyrotoxicosis. All SFD infants should therefore be examined with particular care.

Pathophysiology of SFD

Babies in groups 1 and 2 can be SFD because of abnormalities of uterine shape, or just because they have small parents. Other factors which cause infants to become SFD are those which compromise the transfer of oxygen and nutrients to the fetus:

● Maternal malnutrition

● Maternal illness — urinary tract infection, malaria, severe diabetes

● Maternal hypoxia — cyanotic heart disease, living at high altitude, smoking

● Poor utero-placental function

● Abnormal placentation

● Placental abnormalities

● Pre-eclampsia, placental infarction

   In addition to these obvious disorders, SFD, like prematurity, shows a social class gradient, presumably for much the same reasons.

   Whatever the cause, the end result of all these problems is a fetus who suffers intra-uterine malnutrition and growth retardation. As a result it has poor deposits of glycogen in the myocardium and liver. This causes problems in two situations:

1 During labour. The low glycogen stores compromise the infant's ability to cope with even mild asphyxia by anaerobic glycolysis. Therefore comparatively mild asphyxia can cause sudden intrapartum death.

2 Postnatally. Unless feeding is established immediately, hypoglycaemia develops (Chapter 13).

Obstetric management of SFD infants

Detection

The great problem for the obstetrician is identifying antenatally the infant who is SFD, and therefore at risk from intrapartum asphyxia and intrapartum stillbirth. Even with modern ultrasound techniques, no more than 50% of SFD neonates are correctly identified before delivery.

Antenatal care

If an SFD infant is detected antenatally, then daily monitoring of the fetal movements should be done by the mother from 32 weeks of gestation. If these drop to less than 10 in a 12-hour period, the mother should be seen at once in the maternity hospital. In addition regular checks of the fetal heart rate and its pattern should be made in the antenatal clinic.

Evidence of imminent fetal demise — for example sinister fetal heart-rate decelerations, or the absence of fetal movement, are indications for immediate caesarean section after every effort has been made by ultrasound and even fetoscopic examination to ensure that the fetus has no lethal malformations.

Intrapartum care

In the presence of lesser degrees of fetal growth retardation detected near term, it is probably unwise to let the pregnancy progress beyond 40 weeks. In some such cases the obstetrician may induce the mother between the 38th and 40th week, and allow a short trial of labour, monitoring the baby very carefully. Any evidence of fetal asphyxia in the labour is then an absolute indication for caesarean section. In other cases, the obstetrician may feel that the fetus is so SFD or lacking in glycogen that it would be unable to withstand even the mild asphyxia of a trial of labour, and he would therefore opt for immediate delivery by caesarean section.

Chapter 13
Care of the Healthy Low Birthweight Infant

Many infants weighing less than 2.5 kg, even a few of those weighing less than 1.0 kg remain asymptomatic during the neonatal period. This chapter describes the care of these infants.

Small for dates infants

Diagnosis

All labour wards and PNWs should have a copy of Table 2.1 (Chapter 2) at the nursing station. Infants who are SFD can then be identified easily, and appropriate steps can be taken.

Most SFD infants weigh between 1.8 and 2.5 kg, and are mature with a gestation greater than 37 weeks. The vast majority of these infants are neither malformed nor overtly ill immediately after delivery, and they should be looked after by their mothers on a PNW. For the small minority who weigh less than about 1.8 kg, NNU care is more appropriate, and their management is that described below for asymptomatic preterm infants.

Problems

Hypothermia

SFD infants are susceptible to hypothermia because they have a large surface area to body weight ratio; their body temperature is likely to fall if they are asphyxiated or become hypoglycaemic. However, even if these complications occur, hypothermia is preventable by ensuring that the baby is adequately wrapped up immediately after delivery and not bathed or left naked on a chilly labour ward.

Once on a PNW, an SFD infant should be dressed in a standard baby gown and hat, and swaddled in a double blanket. With this degree of covering a baby weighing more than 1.8–2.0 kg should easily sustain his body temperature in a cot beside his mother's bed.

102

Hypoglycaemia

All SFD babies are at risk from developing hypoglycaemia (less than 1 mmol/1) during the first 60 hours of life, and the smaller the baby, the earlier this is likely to occur. Irrespective of how well they appear to be, all SFD neonates should have their blood glucose checked by Dextrostix at 2, 6, 12, 24, 36 and 48 hours of age, since this will give ample warning of asymptomatic hypoglycaemia before it progresses to symptomatic neuroglycopenia. Equally important however, in order to prevent even asymptomatic hypoglycaemia occuring, all healthy SFD infants should be started on full-strength milk feeds by 2−4 hours of age, giving 3-hourly feeds totalling 60 ml/kg/24 hours on day 1 and 90 ml/kg/24 hours on day 2. If the infant cannot suck, he should be tube-fed. If the mother wishes to breast-feed this should be encouraged, but in addition to the infant going to the breast regularly during the first 48 hours, he must be complemented with the above volume of formula. Three to five per cent of infants managed in this way will still develop asymptomatic hypoglycaemia but an extra feed is usually all that is required to raise their blood glucose above 1.0 mmol/l The management of the infant who becomes symptomatically hypoglycaemic, or whose asymptomatic hypoglycaemia does not respond to feeding, is described in Chapter 23.

Premature infants

Temperature control

Low birthweight infants, particularly if left naked in single-walled incubators loose heat rapidly by the four standard mechanisms (Chapter 5). Particularly if they are very premature and have a thin skin, they have a very high evaporative heat loss due to transepidermal water loss in the first few days of life.

To keep a preterm infant's body temperature normal without him having to do any metabolic work to generate heat, i.e. keeping him in the so-called neutral temperature range, he should be nursed within the environmental temperatures shown in Fig. 5.5.

Most neonates who weigh <1.4−1.5 kg, even when fully-swaddled and wearing a woolly hat, are unable to sustain their body temperature in the nursery at 24−27°C (75°−80°F), and so they need to be kept in an incubator. By the time they weigh 1.5−1.6 kg, however, most of them can be cot-nursed in a room of 24°C (75°F).

Hypoglycaemia

LBW babies are also prone to hypoglycaemia (less than 1.0 mmol/l) and should therefore have their blood glucose checked by Dextrostix once or twice a day until they are well and an adequate milk intake is established.

Nutrition

Adequate nutrition is particularly important for the VLBW infant (<1.5 kg) because:
1 Glycogen stores are small and fat stores are minuscule.
2 Energy needs may be exaggerated by illness.
3 The developing nervous system may be at particular risk from the effects of starvation.

Timing

Feeding should be started in all asymptomatic preterm infants within 2−4 hours of delivery. Infants less than 1−1.25 kg should start on hourly feeds; by the time they weigh 1.25−1.3 kg they can change to 2-hourly feeds, going to 3-hourly by the time they weigh 1.5−1.6 kg.

How to feed

Well infants should be fed enterally, leaving parenteral feeding for ill babies (Chapter 20). There are several advantages of early use of the gastro-intestinal tract even if the actual quantities of nutrients are small.
1 Feeding stimulates production of gut hormones and facilitates peristalsis.
2 Feeding seems to be essential for adequate villus growth; its absence leads to atrophy.
3 Bile flow and bowel function are stimulated; minimizing hyperbilirubinaemia (p.256).
4 Psychological comfort for the mother to know that her baby is being fed.

Technique

Infants less than 1.5−1.6 kg birthweight usually need to be tube-fed initially. Since oro-gastric tubes have to be passed virtually every feed, naso-gastric tubes are preferred since they can be left *in situ* for several days without disturbing the baby. They have the theoretical hazard of compromizing breathing by obstructing one nostril, but this is rarely a clinical problem. Naso-gastric tubes need careful fixation once inserted. Various techniques are used for administering the milk.

Intra-gastric feeding. This has the advantage of being physiological, but the disadvantage of gastric distension, which may compromise ventilation or lead to regurgitation and aspiration. The feed is often given hourly as an intermittent bolus, but may be given as a continuous infusion using a syringe pump. In general the continuous method is preferred for the smaller babies (<1.25 kg) and the intermittent method for larger ones or those who are at less risk from gastric distension.

Trans-pyloric feeding. Some units use this method routinely for VLBW babies, others employ it only if intra-gastric feeds are not tolerated. The main advantage of this method is that gastric dilatation and the risk of aspiration are lessened or avoided. The disadvantages are:
1 Food bypasses the gastric digestive processes, particularly gastric lipase with resultant malabsorption of fat and poorer weight gain.
2 The tube is harder to place (and replace) than a gastric one.
3 The risk of necrotizing enterocolitis (NEC) may be higher.
Nasojejeunal tubes have to be made of soft silastic to avoid perforating the jejeunum, and may take 24−48 hours to pass the pylorus. There is no need to use them routinely. This method undoubtedly has a place, but is probably best confined to those infants who demonstrate an intolerance to gastric feeding.

Once babies weigh more than 1.5 kg, and occasionally when they are even smaller, they will suck at a bottle or the breast. Even if they cannot suck adequately, they should be tried at the breast, since even licking the nipple helps to sustain a mothers lactation, and is a great morale booster for her.

Position for feeding

An infant's stomach empties better if he is lying on his right side or lying prone. Simply maintaining one of these positions after a feed may convert a baby who is difficult to feed into one who is easy to feed.

In general we aim for the feeding schedules shown in Table 13.1 in

Table 13.1.   Volumes of milk (ml/kg) given to healthy premature or SFD infants.*

Day 1 (of life)	60
Day 2	90
Day 3	120
Day 4	150
Day 10	180
Day 14	200

*In some infants especially SFD, it may be indicated to increase to 220 or 250 ml/kg per day.

babies weighing 1.5−2.5 kg. However, some infants weighing <1.5 kg cannot cope with so rapid an increase, in which case the volume given each day is increased more slowly (Table 13.2).

Which milk

The arguments about which milk is best for babies are outlined in Chapter 8. Since bank breast milk is deficient in protein, calories and several minerals (Table 13.3) it is not appropriate for the long-term feeding of preterm infants. Ideally, therefore, we give healthy preterm infants breast milk expressed by their own mother, which fortuitously has a higher protein and mineral content (Table 13.3). If this is not available there are three alternatives:
1 Pooled breast milk from the bank (Table 13.3).
2 Standard infant formulae (Chapter 8).
3 Special formulae adapted for preterm infants by having a higher protein, mineral and calorie content (Table 13.3).
   If the mother is hoping to establish lactation, use bank breast milk in the short-term until her lactation is established. Bank milk is also the preferred milk for starting enteral feeding in infants less than 1.0−1.25 kg birthweight, in particular those who have had bowel problems such as NEC.
   For preterm infants whose mothers are not planning to breast-feed and provide them with 'mothers own' milk, it is clear that the use of banked breast milk results in slower growth and weight gain, and evidence of vitamin and mineral deficiency. In these babies, if necessary after a short period using bank breast milk to establish enteral feeding, one of the special preterm formulae should be given (Table 13.3).

Table 13.2. Volumes of milk (ml/kg) given to LBW infants recovering from severe neonatal illness.*

Day 1 (of life or from start of feeding)	20
Day 2	40
Day 3	60
Day 4	80
Day 5	100
Day 6	120
Day 7	150

*In general 100 ml/kg provides 281.4 kJ/kg (67 kcal/kg). Therefore to give 420−462 kJ/kg (100−110 kcal/kg) requires 150−165 ml/kg of milk.

Vitamin and mineral supplements

We give all infants who weigh less than 2.0 kg 0.2 mg folic acid daily, and 0.3 ml Abidec (Table 13.4) daily. Infants whose birthweight is less than 1.5 kg receive a further daily supplement of 1000 units of vitamin D and 10 mg of vitamin E until they leave the NNU. These infants may also need supplementary sodium and phosphate if they are fed on any type of breast milk.

Iron supplementation in LBW infants may aggravate the tendency to vitamin E deficiency. For this reason we do not give iron supplements until a neonate weighs more than 2.0 kg, when we start 50 mg of ferrous sulphate daily, given as a single dose.

Weight gain

VLBW infants may take 10−20 days to regain their birthweight, but once they are gaining weight it usually increases at about 150−200 g/week if they receive the volume of milk described in Table 13.2. Otherwise healthy <1.5 kg infants may fail to gain weight at the ideal rate. Various causes for this are:

1 An inadequate protein intake. 150−180 ml/kg/24 hours of breast milk does not provide them with enough protein for normal growth. If the baby cannot tolerate 220−250 ml/kg, the alternatives are:

  a Switch to a preterm formula (p.108).

  b Accept the poor weight gain in exchange for the other benefits of breast milk.

2 Inadequate calorie intake. Bank breast milk is low in fat. The treatment is the same as for a low protein intake.

Table 13.3. Composition of milks used for feeding preterm infants (see Chapter 9 for composition of cow's milk and standard formulae).

	Breast milk			Low birthweight formulae		
	Mature*	Preterm	Bank†	SMA low birthweight	Prematalac	Osterprem
Carboydrate (g/100 ml)	7.4	6.4	7.1	8.6	6.6	7.0
Fat (g/100 ml)	4.2	3.1	2.2	4.4	5.0	4.9
Protein (g/100 ml)	1.1	2.7	1.35	2.0	2.4	2.0
Casein/lactalbumin ratio	2:3	2:3	2:3	2:3	2:3	2:3
Sodium (mmol/l)	6.4	17	4.8	14	26	20
Potassium (mmol/l)	15	17	16	19	24	15
Calcium (mg/100 ml)	35 (8)§	29 (7.25)	28 (7)	75 (19)	67 (16.7)	70 (17.5)
Phosphate (mg/100 ml)	15 (4.9)	13 (4.2)	14 (4.5)	40 (12.9)	53 (17.2)	35 (11.3)
Iron (mg/100 ml)	0.08	0.15	—	0.67	0.65	0.04
Vitamin D (µg/100 ml)	0.01			1.3	1.1	8.0
Cals/100 ml	70	74	54	80	79	80

*i.e. from a woman with established lactation.
†Data from milk which is a mixture of expressed breast milk and milk collected as it drips from the contralateral breast while an infant is suckling (drip breast milk).
§Figures in brackets, values in mmol/l.

Table 13.4.   Abidec (composition/0.6 ml).

Vitamin A	4000 units
Vitamin B₁ (thiamine HCl)	1 mg
Vitamin B₂ (riboflavin)	0.4 mg
Pyridoxine	0.5 mg
Nicotinamide	5 mg
Vitamin C (ascorbic acid)	50 mg
Vitamin D (calciferol)	400 units

3 Metabolic acidaemia. Infants, usually formula-fed, may develop a base deficit $>8-10$ mmol/l due to their inability to excrete hydrogen ions. If their weight gain is poor for several days, they should be treated with oral sodium bicarbonate ($2-4$ mmol/kg/24 hours).
4 Occult urinary infection: (p.181).
5 Anaemia of prematurity (see below).
6 Cold stress. Infants nursed in temperatures below thermoneutrality (p.41) and therefore burning brown fat and calories to sustain body temperature gain weight slowly.

All the other causes of failure to thrive in older infants (p.80) can be sought if the more common causes of failure to thrive have been excluded, but the weight gain remains poor.

Anaemia (see also Chapter 25)

Many VLBW infants (particularly those who weigh <1.5 kg at birth, even though they remain well and receive the vitamin supplements described above) become anaemic with haemoglobin levels of $7.0-8.0$ g/l in the 6th–8th week of life. If they are asymptomatic, no treatment is necessary as the haemoglobin rises spontaneously in the next few weeks. In a few, however, this anaemia causes mild breathlessness and some difficulty with feeding; they should be transfused, as should most infants whose haemoglobin falls to <7 g/l.

Parent–baby contact

Throughout the baby's stay on the NNU it is essential that the parents and siblings are allowed unrestricted access to him for all the reasons given in Chapter 3. If the unit has enough mother and baby rooms the parents should be encouraged to stay with their baby as much as they like.

Cross-infection

This has been covered in detail in Chapter 9. The two points to emphasize where LBW babies are concerned are:
1 The importance of hand washing to minimize infection of babies by staff and to prevent cross infection between babies in the unit.
2 The parents and older siblings are not important vectors of infection in an NNU, unless they have an intercurrent illness (Chapter 9).

Discharge (see also Chapters 3 and 30)

Once a baby is feeding well 3-hourly, and gaining weight steadily, and can sustain his body temperature in a room at 70°C, he can be discharged. This usually occurs when his birthweight is between 1.7 and 2.0 kg. Follow-up should be arranged in specific cases (p.323).

Section V

Chapter 14
Resuscitation and its Sequelae

The change from a fetal aquatic parasitic existence to that of an independent air-breathing baby is usually remarkably smooth, most infants announcing their arrival with a welcome yell. Occasionally there is an ominous silence after birth, the infant lying pale and apparently lifeless. This happens in perhaps 5% of mature babies and considerably more frequently in preterm ones. Everyone who is responsible for such infants must be able to treat them immediately; a whole future life may depend on swift, skilful resuscitation.

Physiological changes

During intra-uterine life the fetus is relatively hypoxic, hypercarbic and acidaemic with respect to the mother. Normal labour is a mildly asphyxial process and increases these differences, but with the onset of adequate respiration the baby quickly establishes normal blood gases (Table 14.1). If, however, there is interference with gas exchange before, during or after birth the baby becomes more hypoxic, hypercarbic and acidaemic, the combined results of which may have many deleterious effects.

Pathophysiology of asphyxia

The problems posed by asphyxia before and after birth have been studied in experimental models of acute total asphyxia in which newborn animals are prevented from breathing immediately after delivery by sealing their heads in a saline-filled bag; the resultant physiological changes are then observed, as are the responses to resuscitation.

Respiratory responses during acute asphyxia

Four phases are recognized:
1 The luckless animal struggles and attempts to 'breathe' for a minute or two.
2 There is a period of *primary* apnoea lasting 2−3 minutes.
3 The animal then proceeds to gasp at fairly regular intervals but with

Table 14.1. Maternal, fetal and early neonatal blood gases.

	Maternal	Fetus onset of labour	Fetus end of labour	Infant 1 hour after birth (p.36)
Oxygen saturation (%)	98.5−99	42	30	90
$P_a O_2$ kPa (mmHg)	13.3 (100)	2.6 (20)	2.2 (16)	10.8 (80)
$P_a CO_2$ kPa (mm Hg)	4.5 (34)	5.9 (44)	6.8 (51)	4.1 (31)
Hydrogen ions nmol/l (pH)	37 (7.43)	49 (7.35)	53 (7.28)	40 (7.40)

decreasing vigour until it reaches the 'last gasp' (5−10 minutes after the onset of asphyxia).

4 The stage of *secondary* or *terminal* apnoea is then reached and the animal will die unless actively resuscitated.

The total time to the last gasp is largely determined by the pH at the onset of asphyxia. Maternal sedation tends to prolong the period of primary apnoea at the expense of gasping time.

Cardiovascular responses

1 Initially, during primary apnoea and the phase of gasping, cardiac output is maintained by systemic vasoconstriction and a rise in blood pressure, with redistribution of the circulation mainly to the brain and myocardium.

2 Pulmonary arteriolar vasoconstriction is potentiated with a continuing right-to-left shunt through fetal channels.

3 In terminal apnoea there is progressive bradycardia and hypotension until cardiac arrest occurs 5−10 minutes after the last gasp. The ability to maintain myocardial function throughout this period of total oxygen lack depends on the cardiac glycogen reserves present in newborn animals including the human.

Blood gases

$P_a O_2$ falls precipitously during the first few minutes of asphyxia. One can calculate that all the body's oxygen will be consumed within 2 minutes. Thereafter anaerobic glycolysis takes over with accumulation of lactic acid. $P_a CO_2$ rises progressively to about 20 kPa (150 mmHg) after 10 minutes of total asphyxia. The mixed metabolic and respiratory acidosis results in a H^+ concentration of about 160 nmol/l (pH 6.8). Plasma potassium concentration rises due to H^+ ions entering the cells when the membrane pumps fail.

Responses to resuscitation

If the experiment is terminated while the animal is in *primary* apnoea the onset of gasping can be facilitated by almost any stimulus. In this situation or if the animal is gasping, recovery occurs spontaneously, as oxygen is breathed in. If the phase of *terminal* apnoea has been reached then the animal will only recover if (a) oxygen is forced into the lungs by IPPV and (b) there is sufficient cardiac activity to allow its uptake. As soon as oxygen enters the tissues P_aO_2 rises, myocardial function improves with restoration of heart rate, tissue perfusion and blood pressure. P_aCO_2 falls with IPPV; respiratory centre activity is heralded by gasping followed by the onset of sustained respiration. Hydrogen ion concentration falls due to the rapid elimination of CO_2 but the metabolic component of the acidaemia is much slower to resolve.

The time between resuscitation and the onset of gasping and spontaneous respiration is directly related to the severity of the preceding asphyxia.

The clinical situation

Although acute experimental asphyxia is a useful model, things are seldom as clear cut in real life. Total intra-uterine asphyxia is rare; far more common are one or more episodes of comparatively brief subtotal asphyxia alternating with periods of partial recovery in which case the fetus becomes hypoxic, acidaemic and glycogen depleted much more gradually. The effects of such repeated attacks may be cumulative and cause depression at birth, or the fetus may partially recover from them and be born in relatively good cardio-respiratory condition but have suffered profound neurological damage during the episodes of asphyxia (Chapter 18).

Risk factors

Neonatal asphyxia can often be anticipated, particularly in the presence of one or more of the factors shown in Table 14.2. Under these conditions the paediatrician should be alerted so that he can be present at the delivery.

Assessment of the infant after birth

The Apgar score (based on 5 simple clinical criteria, Table 14.3) is

Table 14.2. Some risk factors for neonatal asphyxia.

Maternal	Fetal
Eclampsia	Premature labour <35 weeks
Pre-eclampsia	Multiple pregnancy
Hypertension during labour	Intra-uterine growth retardation
Diabetes	Prolapsed cord
Antepartum haemorrhage	Meconium stained liquor
Chronic hypertension or renal disease	Fetal distress from any cause
Heavy sedation	Severe Rhesus isoimmunization
Incoordinate uterine action	Delivery by caesarean section
(drug induced-oxytocin)	Forceps delivery
	Breech delivery

Table 14.3. Apgar score, the 5 criteria are given with a mnemonic.

Score	0	1	2
Appearance (colour of trunk)	White	Blue	Pink
Pulse rate (stethoscope heart rate)	Absent	<100	>100
Gasping (respiratory performance)	Absent	Gasping	Regular/crying
Activity (muscle tone)	Limp	Diminished	Normal with active movement
Reflex response (to pharyngeal catheter)	None	Grimace	Cough/sneeze

widely used to give an overall objective evaluation of the infant's condition at birth. The maximum score is 10 and represents an infant in the best possible condition; a score of 0 is technically a stillbirth. Heart rate and respiratory effort are the most valuable criteria. Although originally designed for use at one minute after delivery, make the first assessment immediately after birth and repeat it at 5 minutes to assess progress and response to resuscitation. A disadvantage of a purely numerical score is that it lends itself to too much guesswork, and it is more valuable to note the individual signs as observed; a numerical score can then easily be derived if needed for statistical or research purposes.

Infants are classified at birth into one of four groups:

1 *In good condition* (Apgar 7–10). Blue or pink, breathing or crying, good heart rate and muscle tone.

2 *In moderate condition* (Apgar 4−6). Blue, breathing inadequately or gasping but with a good heart rate.
3 *In poor condition* (Apgar 1−3). Pale or blue, *apnoeic*, limp, slow heart rate. This will include all babies in terminal apnoea, as well as some in primary apnoea.
4 *Dead* (Apgar 0), but perhaps resuscitatable.

Resuscitation

Equipment

The following should be readily available in all places where infants are likely to be born:
1 Oxygen supply with safety blow off valve set at 30 cmH_2O.
2 Self-inflating bag with its own safety blow off device and appropriate face masks.
3 Adequate suction with catheters for nasopharyngeal suction and smaller sizes (FG 5 and 6) for suction down endotracheal tubes.
4 Infant oropharyngeal airways.
5 Laryngoscope and infant blade (also spare bulb and batteries).
6 Endotracheal tubes (size 3.0 and 2.5 mm).
7 Overhead radiant heat source.
8 Stopwatch or clock.
9 Equipment for umbilical catheterization.
10 Selection of syringes, needles, specimen bottles.
11 Drugs. Base (5% or 8.4% sodium bicarbonate, or 7% THAM), naloxone, 10% calcium gluconate, 1/1000 adrenalin, 10% dextrose, 0.9% saline.

Procedure

1 Before the delivery check that all equipment is functioning correctly.
2 Turn on the overhead heater.
3 Glean any relevant information about the pregnancy and delivery from the mother's notes and labour ward staff.
4 As soon as the infant is delivered dry him and wrap him in a warm towel, leaving his upper half exposed.
5 Make a rapid clinical assessment. Infants in good condition need no resuscitation and should not be sucked out unless there is meconium or blood in the airway.
6 If at all possible obtain a sample of cord blood for acid base analysis. This is the most objective assessment of the degree of fetal asphyxia.

Infants in good condition (see Chapter 6)

Infants in moderate condition

Give oxygen by mask. Stimulate by gently slapping the soles of the feet. Assess progress from heart rate, respiratory effort and colour. If heart rate falls and/or ventilation remains inadequate, proceed to bag and mask ventilation. If no response, intubate and ventilate.

Infants in poor condition

This emergency occurs after about 1% of all births. Calm, efficient action is absolutely vital. Failure to act correctly may result in a dead baby or compromise his whole future by causing or accentuating hypoxic ischaemic brain damage. Proceed immediately to intubation and IPPV (Fig. 14.1). One of three things will happen:
1 Infant gasps, then breathes, heart rate improves, and he becomes pink, all within 2–3 minutes (probable primary apnoea).
2 Heart rate improves, infant becomes pink but remains apnoeic or with inadequate respiration (either terminal apnoea or effects of sedation). Continue IPPV and give naloxone if appropriate.
3 Infant remains bradycardic, limp, pale and apnoeic (secondary apnoea with myocardial failure). Boost cardiac output by external massage + drugs (see below). Consider technical error. Once cardiac output has improved proceed with resuscitation as outlined in Fig. 14.1.

Infants born dead

Make an attempt to resuscitate provided the fetal heart has been heard within 5–10 minutes of delivery; at least two pairs of hands are needed. Immediately start external cardiac massage. Intubate and ventilate. Cannulate the umbilical vein and give 5–10 mmol $NaHCO_3$. If there is no sign of life after 3–4 minutes repeat the $NaHCO_3$ and give 1–2 ml of 10% calcium gluconate and 0.5 ml 1/1000 adrenalin. If this fails give further $NaHCO_3$ and intracardiac adrenalin. Abandon resuscitation after 10 minutes if there is no sign of life.

Drugs in resuscitation

There is no place for respiratory stimulant drugs in resuscitation; the

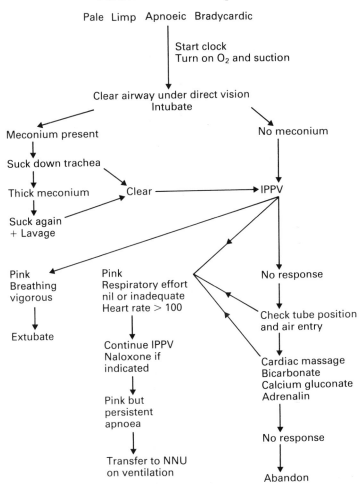

Fig. 14.1. Resuscitation of the severely asphyxiated newborn.

only drug to give is naloxone if the mother has had an opiate within 4 hours of delivery and the infant remains apnoeic despite IPPV. Only give intravenous base ($NaHCO_3$ or THAM) if, after establishing IPPV, the onset of respiration is delayed a further 5–6 minutes.

Evaluation of response to resuscitation

1 Note when the baby becomes pink; once this has happened there is no immediate need for panic.

2 Note time to first gasp and the time to adequate breathing; these give a good indication of the severity of asphyxia.

3 The Apgar score at 5 minutes gives an idea of overall progress.

Techniques for IPPV

Bag and mask

A good fit between mask and face is essential. Hold the jaw forward; occasionally an airway may help. This technique is unlikely to be successful if the baby has never breathed; it may, however, stimulate breathing in the baby in primary apnoea.

Endotracheal intubation (Fig. 14.2)

Have the infant flat or with his neck slightly flexed ('sniffing' position). Hold the laryngoscope in your left hand and slide the blade along the top of the tongue, pushing it away towards the left. Swing the blade upwards and look for the larynx (a triangular-shaped slit) and the epiglottis; the tip of the blade should be in the vallecula. Suck away any mucus or other debris to clear the view. Push the endotracheal tube between the cords with your right hand. Use a 3.0 mm tube for most babies. Establish that the tube is in the correct place by watching chest movement and listening to the air entry over both lungs. Use an inflating pressure of about 30 cmH_2O, rate 30−60/minute. 100% oxygen is generally used.

Meconium

If there was meconium-stained liquor during labour, laryngoscope the baby and aspirate any meconium-stained liquor from the pharynx and trachea during the first minute of resuscitation. If the meconium is thick (like pea soup) suck out the trachea *before* giving IPPV. Sometimes it is necessary to perform bronchial lavage by instilling and then aspirating aliquots of 0.5 ml saline down the trachea.

Failed resuscitation

If the infant's condition does not improve with ventilation consider the following:

1 Bag and mask ventilation is very unlikely to be effective unless the infant has already gasped: proceed to intubation.

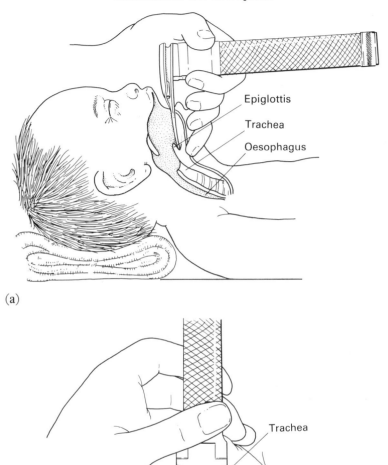

Epiglottis

Trachea

Oesophagus

(a)

Trachea

Vocal chords

(b)

Fig. 14.2. (a) and (b) Technique for intubation. (From Wilkinson and Calvert, 1986.)

2 Tube problems. It may be in the oesophagus, in too far or blocked. Small tubes (<3.0 mm) have a big resistance and allow a large leak. These are diagnosed by noting inadequate chest expansion and treated by correct intubation.

3 Insufficient pressure being applied; check the manometer and watch chest movement; look for leaks.

4 Congenital abnormalities:

  a Diaphragmatic hernia (p.244).

  b Potter's syndrome with lung hypoplasia (p.167).

  c Other rare lung abnormalities are virtually always fatal irrespective of treatment.

5 Blood loss. If the infant is very pale give 10−15 ml/kg of fresh group O Rhesus negative blood.

6 Pneumothorax (p.155); if suggestive, needle the chest and arrange an X-ray.

7 Hydrops fetalis (p.319).

8 Severe RDS (Chapter 15); increase the ventilation pressure.

Care of the asphyxiated infant following resuscitation

Mild asphyxia

Provided the infant is mature, breathing well, pink in air by 10 minutes and is reasonably active, he should stay with his mother (p.93).

Moderate asphyxia

If you are uncertain about the infant's condition admit him to the NNU. Obtain arterial blood for acid-base studies, PCV and blood sugar. If there is severe metabolic acidaemia ($H^+>63$ nmol/l, pH <7.2) consider correction with bicarbonate. Most mature infants will, however, correct this spontaneously by 'blowing off' CO_2. Many babies may be transiently 'jittery', and appear wide-eyed and alert, but make a rapid recovery over the next few hours and can soon be sent to the PNW. Others may have continuing problems and complications (see p.124).

Asphyxia in the low birthweight infant

Low birthweight infants, particularly those <1.5 kg and/or <32 weeks, are at great risk of asphyxia and are often delivered by caesarean section to save them the stress imposed by vaginal delivery, especially in breech presentations. Poor management in this group greatly increases the risk of severe RDS (Chapter 15) and periventricular haemorrhage (p.215). There is a case for intubating all infants <30 weeks at birth before transferring them to the NNU where they can be properly evaluated.

Continuing care of the severely asphyxiated infant

Initial care on admission (i.e. within the first hour)

1 Weigh if possible. Place in a warmed incubator to facilitate observation.
2 Continue IPPV unless obviously breathing well. Give sufficient oxygen to abolish cyanosis.
3 Set up monitoring for heart rate, blood pressure and respiration.
4 Do Dextrostix; if <1.4 mmol/1 check true blood glucose and start intravenous infusion of 10% dextrose.
5 Take blood for baseline acid-base status, electrolytes, culture, PCV and blood count.
6 Do a chest X-ray.
7 If the baby is obviously very sick proceed to umbilical catheterization.
   Further care depends on his progress and the results of the initial investigations.

Respiratory problems

Respiratory distress syndrome in the preterm infant, meconium aspiration in the mature infant and pulmonary haemorrhage are discussed in Chapter 15.

Blood gases

Adjust the inspired oxygen concentration to maintain P_aO_2 at 8–12 kPa (60–90 mmHg). If hypoxaemia persists despite high F_1O_2 consider persistent fetal circulation (p.200). Particularly if brain damage is suspected keep the P_aCO_2 <4.5 kPa (35 mmHg) by IPPV if necessary. If H+ concentration is >63nmol/1 (pH <7.2) and base deficit >10 mmol/1 consider correction with $NaHCO_3$ or THAM.

Anaemia

Always requires correction with transfusion, the lower the Hb the more urgently this should be done. Aim for a PCV of 40% (Hb 13 g/dl).

Hypotension

The myocardial insufficiency associated with asphyxia responds, in most cases, to correction of hypoxia, acidosis, hypoglycaemia and anaemia. Continued hypotension and poor peripheral perfusion indicate myocardial damage or hypovolaemia and it is not always easy to distinguish between these two. Give small aliquots of a volume expander, e.g. PPF 5−10 ml/kg, and observe the response, combine this with frusemide (1 mg/kg), particularly if the heart appears large on X-ray. If this fails use a dopamine infusion (5−20 μg/kg/minute).

Renal problems

Haematuria and albuminuria are not uncommon following asphyxia, and renal ischaemia may lead to oliguria for a few hours and in severe cases, renal failure due to acute tubular and cortical necrosis. The management of renal failure is given on p.281.

Gastro-intestinal problems

Ileus is common after asphyxia and if gut ischaemia has been severe, necrotizing enterocolitis may develop (p.249).

Neurological problems

CNS disturbances occur within 48 hours of the asphyxia and are usually caused by cerebral oedema which may progress to cerebral necrosis; manifestations include:
1 Cerebral irritation shown by a hyperactive infant with a high-pitched cry.
2 Frank convulsions which may also be caused by hypoglycaemia, hypocalcaemia or birth trauma.
3 Apnoeic episodes which may be short convulsions.
4 Abnormal muscle tone. The initial response may be hypotonia and a marked reduction in spontaneous movements and response to stimuli. The hypotonia may:
  a Persist for several days followed by a gradual return to normal.
  b Remain severe with continued convulsions, this carries a grave prognosis.

c Pass into an extensor phase after 12–48 hours with marked hypertonia, opisthotonus or hemisyndromes. This phase may likewise progress to death or there may be a gradual return to normal.

5 Abnormal brain stem responses shown by conjugate deviation of the eyes, pinpoint or fixed dilated pupils and lack of gag reflex.

6 Lack of suck and swallowing reflexes.

7 'Inappropriate' ADH secretion (p.233). This is common to many CNS disorders and is a further indication for fluid restriction.

Management

1 Control convulsions (p.211).

2 Control cerebral oedema by:

a Fluid restriction to 30–60 ml/kg/24 hours.

b Keep $P_a co_2$ about 3.5–4 kPa (25–30 mmHg) to lower cerebral blood flow and hopefully minimize oedema.

c Drugs. Dexamethasone is probably of no value but mannitol (1g/kg) given in the early stages once urine flow has been established may help.

Sequelae

Prognosis is notoriously difficult because there are so many variables.

Good prognostic signs

1 Rapid recovery of the circulation after birth.

2 Spontaneous respiration occurring relatively early and certainly within 20 minutes.

3 Absence of fits, or convulsions lasting less than 48 hours.

4 Rapid return of normal muscle tone and spontaneous movements.

5 Establishment of normal feeding patterns within a week.

Bad prognostic signs

1 Failure to become pink within 5–10 minutes of birth.

2 Failure to make respiratory efforts within 20 minutes of birth.

3 Difficulty in controlling convulsions.

4 Persistent abnormal neurological signs for more than a week (hypotonia, hypertonia, absent primitive reflexes).

5 Failure to establish normal sucking and swallowing within a week.

There is a world of difference between a single short period of acute total asphyxia and repeated episodes which may have a cumulative effect and which are more likely to have long-term consequences. Intellectual impairment following asphyxia is usually combined with cerebral palsy. However, even in the very severe group with an Apgar of 0−1, about 75% of survivors develop normally, 6% are severely handicapped, 4% are deaf and the remainder have a variety of problems such as fits, squints, language difficulties and 'hyperactivity'.

References

Wilkinson, A. & Calvert, S. (1986) Procedures in neonatal intensive care. In *Textbook of Neonatology*, N.R.C. Roberton (ed.), Churchill Livingstone, Edinburgh. pp.817−35.

Further reading

Roberton, N.R.C. (1986) Resuscitation of the newborn. In *Textbook of Neonatology*, N.R.C. Roberton (ed.), Churchill Livingstone, Edinburgh. pp.193−203.

Chapter 15
Respiratory Problems in the Newborn

Respiratory problems are the 'bread and butter' of neonatology. They constitute about 75% of the illnesses in this age group, principally in the premature infant. However, not all respiratory symptoms are due to primary lung disease; congenital heart disease, infection, and CNS disturbance can present as respiratory distress as can some congenital malformations.

Respiratory distress in the neonatal period

Within four hours of birth

Infants may show one or more of the following symptoms:
- Tachypnoea (>60/minute)
- Retractions (subcostal, sternal or intercostal)
- Grunting on expiration
- Cyanosis

The possible underlying causes for the distress are:
- Hyaline membrane disease (HMD) or respiratory distress syndrome (RDS) (see below)
- Transient tachypnoea of the newborn (TTN) (p.149)
- Congenital pneumonia (p.178)
- Persistent fetal circulation (p.200)
- Meconium aspiration (p.149)
- Metabolic acidosis following asphyxia (with or without aspiration)
- Pneumothorax or pneumomediastinum (p.151)
- Pulmonary haemorrhage (p.157)
- Congenital abnormalities:
  a Potter's syndrome (p.167).
  b Diaphragmatic hernia (p.244).
  c Congenital heart disease (Chapter 17).
  d Hydrops fetalis (p.319).
  e Rare congenital abnormalities of the airways and lungs (p.165).
- Haematological causes (Chapter 25):
  a Severe anaemia.
  b Polycythaemia.

After four hours of age

Although several rare intrathoracic malformations (all easily diagnosed on CXR) may present after four hours of age, respiratory symptoms in such infants are usually due either to the pulmonary oedema of heart failure (p.193) or pneumonia (p.178). Differential diagnosis is rarely a problem.

Respiratory distress syndrome (RDS) or hyaline membrane disease (HMD)

These two terms are used almost synonymously to describe a form of respiratory distress that is often evident at birth, and always within 4 hours.

Clinical features of RDS

The infant shows the following characteristic signs:

Retractions. In response to the underlying atelectasis, the infant's strenuous efforts to breathe result in subcostal and intercostal retractions; if severe the sternum may appear almost to reach the backbone.

Tachypnoea (RR >60/minute). This very non-specific sign is seen in other forms of respiratory distress. Very premature or very sick infants may lack sufficient respiratory drive and hence have respiratory rates <40. The same is true for drug-depressed infants.

Grunting. A characteristic moan on expiration is produced by the infant expiring against a partially closed glottis and thus attempting to keep his lungs expanded.

Cyanosis. All babies with RDS become hypoxic (p.131) but clinical cyanosis should not occur because the infant should be receiving sufficient oxygen (see p.136).

General clinical picture

The infant tends to lie inert and frequently adopts a 'frog like' posture; he may be oedematous. The heart rate shows little beat-to-beat variation (usually 120−130/minute). Auscultation of the lungs may reveal reduced air entry but this is highly subjective, a few fine crepitations may be heard. There is oliguria and often delay in passing meconium; oral feeds are not tolerated.

These symptoms are common to other causes of neonatal respiratory distress but the commonest cause is surfactant deficient RDS. Pulmonary histology in such neonates shows HMD, which refers to a characteristic histological picture of eosinophilic 'membranes' lining the alveolar ducts.

RDS is far and away the commonest cause of respiratory distress; the incidence varying inversely with GA (Fig. 15.1). Although it is now rare for infants to die from uncomplicated RDS the disease and its complications are still the leading cause of death in the neonatal period (Chapter 2).

Aetiology and pathogenesis (Fig. 15.2)

Deficiency of surfactant is the fundamental aetiological factor. At the moment of birth an enormous amount of surfactant is needed to coat all the terminal airways, an area of approximately 5 m². A relative lack of surfactant at birth may occur for one or more of the following reasons:

1 Immaturity of its synthetic pathways.

2 Interference with its production by pre- or postnatal asphyxia.

3 Qualitative surfactant abnormalities, e.g. failure to produce phosphatidylglycerol (see below).

4 Impaired release onto the alveolar surface.

5 Necrosis and desquamation of the alveolar lining cells which produce the surfactant.

Besides prematurity, the other clinical factors that have traditionally

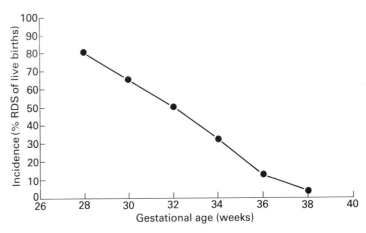

Fig. 15.1. Incidence of RDS related to gestational age (adapted from Roberton, 1986).

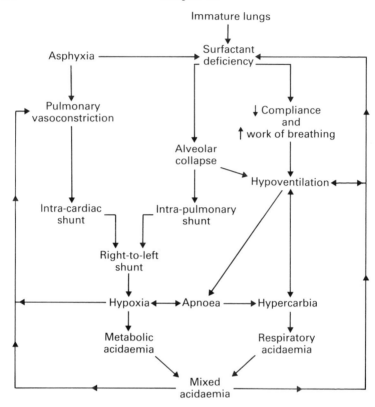

Fig. 15.2. Aetiology and pathogenesis of RDS.

been associated with RDS include intrapartum or neonatal asphyxia (factor 2 above), maternal diabetes (perhaps due to factor 3 above) and caesarean section (this is probably more related to the *indication* for it — or whether it is done pre- or post-labour). Delayed clearance of pulmonary fluid leading to impaired release of surfactant may be responsible for the transient form of respiratory distress (TTN p.149).

Pathophysiology (Figs 15.2 and 15.3)

Failure to establish an adequate alveolar lining layer of surfactant leads to lack of lung expansion after birth and progressive *collapse* of the terminal airspaces. Lung compliance and FRC are decreased and the work of breathing is increased. Initially minute ventilation is maintained by increased frequency, particularly in larger infants. Eventually, however, the progressive decrease in lung volume results

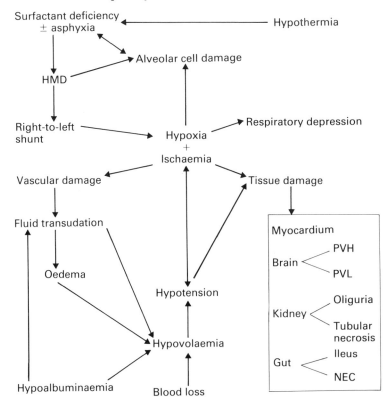

Fig. 15.3. Pathophysiology and complications of RDS.

in alveolar hypoventilation and CO_2 retention, particularly in smaller infants. Hypoventilation further depresses the release of surfactant.

Hypoxia

This is the hallmark of RDS and results from intra-pulmonary shunting usually with a smaller extra-pulmonary shunt through the foramen ovale and ductus arteriosus sustained by the high pulmonary arterial pressure of hypoxia (p.39). *Intrapulmonary shunting* occurs when pulmonary capillary blood flows past alveoli that are either totally non-ventilated (ventilation/perfusion ratio=0), or through partially aerated ones (ventilation/perfusion ratio < 1). The hypoxia, if allowed to persist, can then produce multiple and interrelated derangements:

1 *Metabolic acidaemia:* due to lactic acid accumulation from anaerobic glycolysis; combined with hypoxia this leads to further pulmonary hypertension.

2 *Respiratory depression:* hypoventilation (p.30), hypercarbia and apnoea which further accentuate the hypoxia. The respiratory acidaemia may then contribute to pulmonary hypertension.

3 *Hypotension:* which may also be due to blood loss. It leads to hypoperfusion of all organs and further tissue hypoxia and acidaemia. Hypotension with or without hypovolaemia can have secondary effects on many organ systems:

- Kidney: oliguria and reduced hydrogen ion excretion
- Brain: hypoxic/ischaemic injury, PVH (Chapter 18)
- Gastro-intestinal tract: reduced peristalsis and inability to absorb feeds; necrotizing enterocolitis (p.249)
- Liver: reduced bilirubin conjugation (jaundice) and reduced production of clotting factors
- Skin: a peculiar 'brawny' hard oedema (sclerema)

The increased capillary permeability present in premature infants combined with hypoxic damage to capillary endothelial cells leads to transudation of fluid into the interstital space resulting in generalized oedema (including pulmonary), further aggravating hypoxia and hypotension.

Morbid anatomy of RDS

The lungs of infants who die from RDS appear solid and liver-like.

Histology

The term HMD describes the extensive eosinophilic 'membranes' that line dilated alveolar ducts, the terminal airspaces (the future alveoli) being completely collapsed. There is extensive necrosis and desquamation of the epithelial cells; surfactant is almost completely lacking. After about 3 days some regeneration of the alveolar epithelium starts to occur together with the reappearance of surfactant.

Radiology of RDS

The classic chest X-ray of RDS shows a 'ground glass' or a reticulogranular pattern due to the multiple areas of atelectasis (Fig. 15.4a); if the latter is more extensive the lungs appear as a 'white-out' with the heart shadow being virtually indiscernible (Fig. 15.4b). There is also a characteristic 'air bronchogram', the air-filled bronchi contrasting with the underlying atelectasis (see Fig. 15.4a).

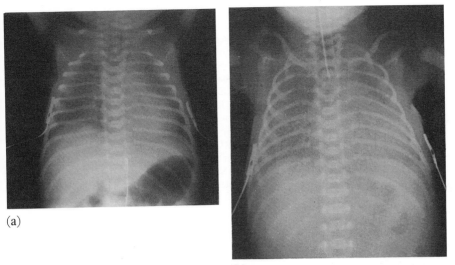

(a)

(b)

Fig. 15.4. (a) RDS showing 'ground glass' appearance and air bronchogram.
(b) RDS showing a 'whiteout' of the lung fields.

Differential diagnosis

The most important other conditions to consider are given on p.127. The history, GA, physical findings and chest X-rays (Table 15.1) will sort out most of them. In general, dyspnoea in a preterm infant is due to RDS, whereas in a more mature infant any diagnosis is possible. The non-pulmonary causes of dyspnoea, e.g. acidaemia and anaemia must be excluded.

Clinical course of RDS

Provided the infant is born in good condition, receives adequate postnatal support and does not suffer any major complications (p.135), the natural history of the disease is one of gradual improvement after 2–3 days and a full recovery over the next 3–7 days. One may broadly classify the disease as mild, moderate, severe, or complicated.

Mild RDS. Affected infants are generally larger and more mature (>34 weeks, >2.0 kg). They are tachypnoeic (>60), grunt loudly but

Table 15.1.   Radiological and clinical features of different forms of respiratory distress.

Condition	X-ray and differential diagnosis
RDS	Reticulo-granular pattern ('ground glass') Air bronchogram May be complete 'white-out'
TTN (p.149)	'Streaky' ling fields Fluid in fissures
Pneumonia (p.178)	Coarse patchy infiltrates. May be indistinguishable from RDS
Meconium aspiration (p.149)	Streaky infiltrates, overexpansion initially. Later coarse infiltrates. History very helpful
Persistent fetal circulation (PFC) (p.200)	Lung fields oligaemic despite profound hypoxia. X-ray and ECG may be virtually normal. Echocardiogram excludes cyanotic heart disease
Pneumothorax (p.151)	Obvious on frontal view
Pneumomediastinum (p.151)	Halo of air round heart on frontal view; air anteriorly on lateral
Congenital heart disease (Chapter 17)	Large heart, lung fields may be oligaemic. ECG and echocardiogram usually diagnostic
Pulmonary hypolasia (p.167)	Very small lungs and rib cage; oligohydramnios
Diaphragmatic hernia (p.244)	Bowel in chest

do not have pronounced retractions. Their oxygen requirements rarely exceed 60% and, by definition, they do not need ventilatory assistance. They spontaneously improve after about 2 days. This group merges imperceptibly into those classed as having transient tachypnoea of the newborn (TTN, p.149).

Moderate RDS. These infants tend to be slightly less mature (31–34 weeks, 1.5–2.0 kg). They manifest all the classic symptoms; oxygen requirements exceed 60% and they may need continuous positive airway pressure (CPAP, p.141) or even a short period (12–48 hours) of ventilation. A gradual recovery ensues from about the third day.

Severe RDS. These infants are generally the most immature (<30 weeks, <1.5 kg). They have pronounced retractions and may not be tachypnoeic but may become apnoeic. High oxygen concentrations are required and they commonly have CO_2 retention; they need ventilation, often for many days; recovery generally starts between 3–7 days. It is now rare for such infants to die, although their recovery can be prolonged and they may develop chronic lung disease (p.158).

Complicated RDS. These infants are most often those in the severe group. The complications can be divided into two broad groups (which are not mutually exclusive); firstly, those that are integral to the pathophysiology (p.130) and others which are true complications of the treatment given. The least mature infants tend to have the most complications and hence a more protracted course.

Complications related to pathophysiology

1 Pneumomediastinum or pneumothorax secondary to large negative pressures produced by the infant struggling to breathe; these may also be iatrogenic (see below).
2 Periventricular haemorrhage (PVH) secondary to episodes of asphyxia and marked swings in blood pressure (p.215).
3 Renal failure secondary to ischaemic renal damage (p.279).
4 Necrotizing enterocolitis (NEC) secondary to gut ischaemia (p.249).
5 Patent ductus arteriosus (PDA p.139).
6 Hypoxic/hypotensive/ischaemic CNS disorders (HIE, PVL; p.219).

True complications

1 Air leaks secondary to assisted ventilation (p.152); pneumomediastinum, pneumothorax, pulmonary interstitial emphysema, pneumopericardium, pneumoperitoneum, subcutaneous emphysema, systemic air embolism). These may all predispose to PVH.
2 Fluid overload leading to patent ductus arteriosus (PDA) and heart failure.
3 Under-hydration leading to hypovolaemia, hypotension and hypernatraemia.
4 Blood loss secondary to blood sampling or disconnected catheters.
5 Metabolic problems in glucose, sodium, potassium, calcium homeostasis (Chapter 19).
6 Infection introduced from indwelling endotracheal tubes (p.178), catheters, etc.
7 Bronchopulmonary dysplasia (BPD; p.158).
8 Oxygen toxicity, including retinopathy of prematurity (p.317).

Initial management on admission

1 Quickly weigh the baby (even if he has an endotracheal tube); a baseline weight is invaluable for calculating appropriate fluid and electrolyte therapy.

2 Put him in a warmed incubator; the ones with overhead heaters make access and procedures much easier and safer. Examine him, remembering to take the BP.

3 Give sufficient oxygen to abolish cyanosis.

4 Set up continuous ECG monitoring.

5 Obtain blood for gases, blood group, blood count, PCV and culture. This may be either from an umbilical or peripheral artery (see below). Venous blood is adequate for everything except blood gases.

6 Insert an umbilical artery catheter (UAC) if it seems likely that the baby will require monitoring for more than 12−24 hours.

7 Start the baby on i.v. antibiotics (given through the catheter or a peripheral drip (see p.140 for reasons).

8 X-ray the chest and abdomen not only to establish the diagnosis but also to check the position of the UAC.

9 Re-assess the situation in the light of clinical progress and results of the preliminary investigations.

Oxygen therapy

Oxygen is the cornerstone of therapy for RDS but it is vital to steer correctly between the Scylla of hypoxia and the Charybdis of oxygen toxicity. The aim is to keep arterial P_{O_2} at 8−12 kPa (60−90 mmHg). Levels below 6−8 kPa (45−60 mmHg) may lead to serious hypoxia and all the associated dangers. On the other hand, hyperoxaemia carries a risk of retinopathy of prematurity (ROP) in the very premature infant <30 weeks (p.317). Very high *inspired* oxygen concentrations (>90%) are toxic to the lungs and should therefore be avoided.

Giving oxygen (except at concentrations <30%) directly into the incubator is ineffective and dangerous because marked fluctuations occur when it is opened for nursing care and because it is almost impossible to obtain concentrations >60%; it should, therefore, always be given into a headbox if concentrations >30% are being used and must always be warmed and humidified. It is essential to monitor the concentration continuously with an accurate analyser. When assisted ventilation is being used, air and oxygen should pass through an accurate mixer displaying the concentration.

Monitoring blood gases

Blood is taken preferably from an indwelling arterial line using one of the following techniques:

Umbilical arterial catheters (UAC). These are easy to insert and allow for repeated painless blood sampling; they can also be used for fluid and antibiotic administration. Infused fluids should be heparinized (2 u/ml). Catheters with a continuous reading oxygen electrode at their tip should be used. Insert a UAC in any infant <1.5 kg with respiratory distress; it can always be removed if the baby improves rapidly. With larger infants, unless they are very sick one can always afford to wait and see for a few hours.

Peripheral arterial lines. The radial, posterior tibial and dorsalis pedis arteries can all be cannulated, but they must not be used for intravenous therapy. The cannulae are kept patent by a slow infusion (0.5−1.0 ml/hour) of heparinized (2 u/ml) normal saline.

Transcutaneous (Po_2 and Pco_2) monitoring is now possible using heated skin electrodes. This technique is very useful in well perfused babies but can be totally unreliable if the skin is not well perfused (hypotension, peripheral shutdown), or if the baby has a thick skin. The values obtained must always be checked at least twice daily against arterial blood gases in infants at risk from ROP.

Umbilical venous catheters (UVC). It is always possible to insert a UVC. They can sometimes be useful for infusing fluids and sampling if a UAC is not feasible), but should not be used for P_aO_2 measurements.

If cannulae cannot be inserted periodic arterial punctures are done. Capillary samples from a warmed heel can be used for measuring H^+, Pco_2 and base deficit, but capillary Po_2 is totally unreliable.

Continuing management

1 Careful observation of the clinical state (colour, retractions, muscle tone and vital signs).
2 Minimal handling: small and sick infants tolerate handling very poorly, even nappy changing can produce alarming downward swings in P_aO_2 (Fig. 15.5).
3 Keep the infant in a neutral thermal environment to minimize heat losses (p.40). Overhead radiant heaters make intensive care easier but cause large transepidermal fluid losses.
4 Fluid and electrolyte balance. Start with 10% dextrose at 60 ml/kg

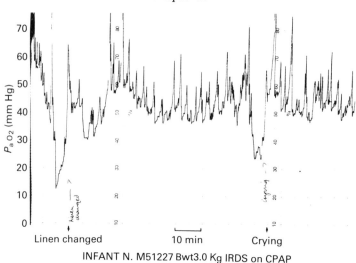

Fig. 15.5. Changes in P_aO_2 (mmHg) with handling and crying. (From Roberton, 1986, with permission.)

(Chapter 19) and usually keep <90 ml/kg until there is a spontaneous diuresis on the second to fourth day which heralds an improvement in lung function. Keep plasma albumin >20 g/l with infusions of plasma or albumin.

5 Nutrition (Chapter 20). Milk feeding should usually be delayed until there are some signs of recovery. Larger infants (>1.5 kg) can tolerate relative starvation (i.v. dextrose alone) for 4−5 days but smaller ones should be started on parenteral nutrition after 2−3 days.

6 Keep the PCV >40% with blood transfusions.

Blood gas and acid base homeostasis

Oxygen. Aim to keep the P_aO_2 at 8−12 kPa (60−90 mmHg) although levels of 6−8 kPa (45−60 mmHg) are acceptable under some circumstances.

CO_2. Aim for a P_aCO_2 of 5−7 kPa (37.5−52.5 mmHg). A level of 8 kPa (60 mmHg) is acceptable provided the hydrogen ion concentration is below 60 nmol/1 (pH >7.25) particularly in larger or older babies not at risk from PVH (p.216).

Hydrogen ions. Should be 35−55 nmol/l (pH 7.3−7.45).

Base deficit. This gives a measure of the metabolic component of any acid base disturbance. By definition it is normally 0 with a normal range between +5 and −5 mmol/l. Values below −10 mmol/l should be corrected with intravenous base. The dose of base is calculated by the following formula:

Dose in mmol = base deficit in mmol/l × body weight (kg) × 0.3.

$NaHCO_3$ is usually used but should never be infused faster than 0.5 mmol/minute. It is sometimes preferable to use THAM (an organic buffer than does not contain sodium); 7% THAM has about the same pH correcting effect as 5% $NaHCO_3$. Remember, however, that metabolic acidaemia is often an indication of tissue hypoxia and therefore the remedy is to improve oxygenation and/or correct hypovolaemia, hypotension or anaemia.

Cardiovascular management

Small, sick babies often have a heart rate fixed at about 120−130/minute.

Bradycardia (<100) indicates hypoxic/apnoeic episodes or CNS malfunction and is potentially serious if prolonged for more than a few minutes.

Tachycardia (>180) may have many causes. Always consider heart failure, fluid overload, anaemia, sepsis, or drugs (e.g. theophylline).

Blood pressure. Maintain the systolic BP above 40 mmHg by colloid infusions if the PCV is >40−45% and by fresh whole blood if the PCV is below 40%. Once any volume deficits have been corrected maintain BP with a dopamine infusion (5−20 μg/kg/minute).

Ductus arteriosus (PDA)

A large and significant left−right shunt through the ductus develops after the first few days in 20−30% of infants <1.5 kg ventilated for RDS. The incidence can be kept to a minimum by meticulous control of the fluid balance. A PDA leads to a torrential pulmonary blood flow, pulmonary oedema and heart failure (p.193); if detected in a baby with RDS it should always be treated (p.194).

Bacteriological and antibiotic management

Cultures of skin, nose, throat and gastric aspirate as well as blood are taken on admission in all babies with any type of respiratory distress. It is impossible to distinguish between respiratory distress due to RDS and that due to sepsis, and both problems may coexist. Although the group B Streptococcus is the commonest culprit, many other organisms can be involved. Therefore put *all* babies with symptoms of respiratory distress on penicillin. A second antibiotic (e.g. gentamicin or a suitable third generation cephalosporin) is added if:

1 There has been prolonged rupture of membranes.
2 The mother is ill or known to be colonized with a potential pathogen.
3 The baby is hypotensive or looks very sick.
4 Initial tests on the baby suggest infection, e.g. positive Gram stain on gastric aspirate or the white count is very low ($<6 \times 10^9/1$; [6000/mm^3]).
5 Initial cultures are positive.
6 Ventilation is needed.

Antibiotics can be discontinued after 48 hours if the initial cultures are sterile and the baby is progressing well.

Ventilatory management of RDS

The indications for conservative management (head box oxygen) rather than CPAP or IPPV depend on birthweight, GA and subsequent clinical progress.

Indications for conservative management

1 Infants >1.5 kg who are well in $<60\%$ oxygen to start with and who maintain adequate blood gases ($P_aO_2 >8$ kPa [60 mmHg], $P_aCO_2 <8$ kPa [60 mmHg], $H^+ = <60$ nmol/l [pH >7.22]). Babies >2 kg seldom need ventilatory assistance and in any case tolerate CPAP badly. They may need $80-90\%$ O_2 but usually keep reasonable blood gases although they may need supplementary O_2 for a week or more.
2 Infants <1.5 kg, who are in good condition at or shortly after birth and who remain well in $<40\%$ O_2 with little or no CO_2 retention and have minimal signs and X-ray changes, come to no harm from a period of conservative treatment and usually recover without further intervention.

Indications for CPAP (see below)

1 Infants 1.5−2.0 kg whose P_aO_2 falls to <8 kPa (60 mmHg) in 60% O_2, particularly during the first 3 days. P_aCO_2 need not be considered.
2 Infants 1.5−2.0 kg who, despite maintaining satisfactory blood gases, have deepening retractions or transient periods of apnoea.
3 Infants <1.5 kg with RDS who are breathing well in less than 50% oxygen. CPAP frequently improves the oxygenation of these babies and their retractions become less obvious.

Indications for IPPV (see below)

1 All babies who require IPPV for resuscitation at birth and who never establish regular spontaneous respiration. IPPV should be continued in such cases until the RDS resolves.
2 All babies who fail to come round immediately from cyanotic/ apnoeic episodes.
3 Babies >1.5 kg who deteriorate on CPAP in >80% oxygen (P_aO_2 <8 kPa [60 mmHg], P_aCO_2 >8 kPa [60 mmHg], H^+ = >60 nmol/l [pH <7.22]) or who have multiple apnoeic attacks.
4 Babies under 1.5 kg. The threshold for ventilating these infants is lower than for larger ones; there may be a case for ventilating all of them from birth unless they are clearly vigorous and without signs of respiratory distress. Do not hesitate too long before ventilating them.

Techniques for ventilatory assistance

Continuous positive airways pressure (CPAP). This is further extension of the 'grunt' mechanism (p.128) by which the spontaneously breathing infant attempts to hold his lungs inflated during expiration. This is accomplished by applying a positive pressure to the upper airway in the following ways:
1 Through an endotracheal tube (also useful during weaning from IPPV).
2 Through a face mask applied tightly over the baby's nose and mouth (unsatisfactory due to the high incidence of complications).
3 Using a box over the infant's head with a neck seal; this method is now very little used.
4 Through nasal prongs. Some centres use a prong in each nostril. We use a single prong (a short, soft endotracheal tube) inserted 2 cm into the nostril. Most neonatal ventilators now have a circuit for giving

CPAP by tube or prong. Whenever giving CPAP the following rules apply:

1 Do not exceed a pressure of 10 cmH_2O (usually 4—7 cmH_2O).
2 Keep an open-ended naso-gastric tube in the stomach to act as a vent.
3 Keep the prong clear by suction.

Intermittent positive pressure ventilation (IPPV). Ventilating infants with RDS presents unique difficulties because:
1 The lungs in RDS are very 'stiff'.
2 There are extensive areas of atelectasis.
3 There is frequently a regional and changing pattern of mismatch between ventilation and perfusion.
4 Pulmonary damage from ventilation therapy is very common (pneumothorax p.155, BPD p.158).

To overcome these problems:
1 Always use the lowest pressures and rates compatible with normal blood gases (p.36).
2 Avoid peak pressures >30 cmH_2O if at all possible — accepting compromise blood gas values (e.g. P_aO_2 of 6—8 kPa, P_aCO_2 of 7—9 kPa).
3 Use high mean airway pressures rather than high peak pressures to obtain satisfactory oxygenation. This can be achieved in various ways by:
  a Increasing the inspiration/expiration ratio sometimes to 2:1.
  b Increasing positive end expiratory pressure (PEEP).
4 Increase peak inflation pressure >30 cmH_2O only as a last resort.
5 Use fast rates (60—150/minute). This may be particularly valuable if the infant's own spontaneous rate and inspiratory time can be matched by the ventilator.
6 Consider drugs — tolazoline, pancuronium (p.145).

Ventilators

Most neonatal ventilators are of the constant flow/pressure limited, time-cycled type. New refinements are constantly taking place but the following characteristics are essential:
● Rates 0—150 with display
● Maximum inflating pressure 10—60 cmH_2O
● PEEP 2—10 cm
● I/E ratio 3:1—1:10
● Good humidification

Ventilator management

For most babies ventilated for RDS, initial ventilator settings should be:
- Rate 40–60/minute
- Peak pressure 20–25 cmH$_2$O
- PEEP 3–5 cmH$_2$O
- Inspiration/expiration ratio 1:1
- O$_2$ concentration 60–80%

Subsequent changes in these settings are based on the results of blood gas analyses. These should be checked after IPPV is set up and then 4-hourly or more often if rapid changes are occuring; the following are guidelines for the action to be taken.

Hyperoxaemia. Reduce F$_1$O$_2$ in 5% steps.

Hypoxia. Consider cause (e.g. pneumothorax, hypotension). Increase F$_1$O$_2$ in steps to 90%. Increase mean airway pressure (see above). Consider tolazoline or pancuronium (p.145).

Hypocapnia. Reduce peak pressure and/or rate.

Hypercapnia. Consider cause (? pneumothorax). Increase rate. Reduce PEEP (if normoxaemic). Increase peak pressure. Consider pancuronium.

Metabolic acidaemia. Correct hypotension and anaemia, consider infection and PVH. If base deficit >10 mmol/l, give intravenous base (p.139).

   In practice, these changes are seldom seen in isolation so that frequently a trial and error approach is needed to find the correct ventilator settings.

Nursing management. Ventilation settings and clinical observation (Fig. 15.6) are recorded by the nursing staff every 30–60 minutes. They should turn the baby every 2–3 hours and suck out his endotracheal tube every 4–6 hours.

Sudden deterioration on ventilator ('collapse')

Everyone concerned in neonatal intensive care should know what to do:

Chapter 15

INFANT VENTILATOR CHART

Name: _____   Hospital number: _____

	Check and/or record[*]	DATE _____ Record time in top box								
BABY	Time									
Colour	1 hourly									
Heart rate	1 hourly									
Blood pressure	4 hourly									
Peripheral circ.	1 hourly									
Temperature	4 hourly									
Chest movement	1 hourly									
Muscular activity	1 hourly									
Posture	1 hourly									
VENTILATOR										
Insp. pressure	1 hourly									
Exp. pressure	1 hourly									
Rate	1 hourly									
Insp. time	1 hourly									
Insp/Exp ratio	1 hourly									
Flow rate	1 hourly									
O_2 concentration	1 hourly									
Humidifier level	2 hourly									
Check tubes	1 hourly									
Suction trachea[†]										
Suction pharynx	2 hourly									
OTHER OBSERVATIONS										
P_aO_2 (electrode)	1 hourly									
Transcut. PO_2	1 hourly									
Incubator temp	4 hourly									
IV fluid given	1 hourly									
Dextrostix	6 hourly									
Blood taken										
Other										

[*] The frequency of observations is that for a baby in a relatively stable condition.

[†] The frequency of suction is individualized.

Fig. 15.6. A ventilator chart.

1 Check whether positive pressure is being applied; if not there must be a fault in the ventilator circuit.

2 Check whether the baby's chest is moving. If not the tube may be displaced or blocked. Suck the tube out; if not blocked, hand-ventilate. If there is still no movement extubate, suck out the trachea and replace the tube.

3 If the chest is moving, increase F_IO_2 and consider pneumothorax (p.155). Increase the inflation pressure.

Tolazoline

This drug has been used for its dilator effect on the pulmonary circulation causing a fall in pulmonary blood pressure, reversing the right-to-left shunt and thus relieving hypoxia. It is given as a bolus dose of $1-2$ mg/kg intravenously; if an effect is observed it can be infused continuously at $1-2$ mg/kg/hour. Systemic vasodilation may also occur causing systemic hypotension, hence the BP may have to be maintained with plasma infusions or dopamine.

Indication. Severe hypoxia (P_aO_2 <5 kPa in 95% O_2) which persists despite adequate IPPV and relatively normal CO_2 and pH measurements. The drug is most effective when given in the first 24 hours.

Pancuronium

The arguments for paralysis are that it makes IPPV much easier to control and that it may prevent air leaks by abolishing any tendency for the infant to breathe out during the ventilator's inspiratory phase. Consider the use of pancuronium under the following circumstances:

1 The infant 'fights the ventilator' despite manipulating the inspiratory time and rate to get him to synchronize with the ventilator; this not only increases the risk of pneumothorax, but may also perpetuate hypoxia and is paticularly likely with infants >2.0−2.5 kg.

2 When using high peak pressures (>30 cmH_2O).

3 Where a pneumothorax or PIE has already developed.

Give pancuronium $100-200$ μg/kg $3-4$ hourly; the disadvantages are:

1 That higher inflating pressures may, in fact, be needed.

2 The absence of muscle tone leads to venous stasis and peripheral oedema.

3 Enteral nutrition is virtually impossible.

4 The sight of a completely flaccid, unresponsive infant is upsetting for the parents.

Complications of IPPV for RDS

- Pneumothorax, PIE (p.151)
- Brochopulmonary dysplasia (p.158)
- Pneumonia/infection (p.178)
- Subglottic stenosis (p.165)

The management of each of these complications is described elsewhere. Individually or together these complications may prove fatal or prolong the period during which oxygen is required, with or without IPPV, to weeks or months.

Nutrition

After 2−3 days on a ventilator start enteral or parenteral nutrition in addition to the dextrose electrolyte mixture (Chapter 20).

Weaning from the ventilator

It can be difficult to 'wean' infants off the ventilator and long periods of ventilation may be needed at rates of 1−15 breaths/minute (the so-called intermittent mandatory ventilation, IMV).

The first priority is to get pressures below 26−28 cmH$_2$O and then to reduce the F$_I$O$_2$ to less than 80%. Then reduce peak inflation pressures in steps of 1−2 cm to 20−22 cmH$_2$O. Then the rate is gradually reduced. Once oxygen requirements have fallen to 30−40% and the baby is normocapnic at inflation pressures of about 20 cmH$_2$O and rates of 20/minute or less, limit the inspiratory time to 0.5 seconds or less (i.e. IMV). Then:

1 When the rate has been reduced to 5−10/minute or less, wean the baby onto CPAP through the ETT at pressures of 4−5 cmH$_2$O.

2 After a trial on very slow rates or ETT CPAP alone, extubate and put the baby on nasal CPAP also at pressures of 4−5 cmH$_2$O or into a headbox. Always stop oral feeds for 12−24 hours after extubation.

3 Be ready to reventilate if these procedures are not well tolerated (rising $P_a$co$_2$, apnoea, etc.). Infants >1.5 kg usually come off quite easily but in smaller babies several attempts and prolonged periods of IMV may be needed.

Theophylline

This drug, acting as a central respiratory stimulant, can be a very valuable aid to weaning from the ventilator. It is given intravenously (as aminophylline) or orally in a loading dose of 6 mg/kg, followed by 1.5–2.0 mg/kg 6-hourly. Therapy should be monitored by blood levels (therapeutic range 27–83 μmol/l [5–15 mg/dl]).

Extubation problems

Nutrition. The nutrition of some infants is still borderline when they are extubated; when combined with several episodes of stopping feeding after extubation, this may produce a puny little baby incapable of sustaining spontaneous respiration. In such cases, reventilate for 7–10 days, while establishing adequate nutrition orally or parenterally.

Atelectasis. Retained secretions may block large parts of the bronchial tree after extubation. This can be minimized by post-extubation positioning and physiotherapy, but may require endobronchial suction or re-intubation and ventilation.

Exhaustion. Infants <1.5 kg, in the hours following extubation, may breathe well but with increasing dyspnoea, a metabolic acidaemia and eventually CO_2 retention and hypoxia. They should be ventilated for a further 24–48 hours, before making another attempt to wean them.

Stridor. Mild stridor following extubation is not too uncommon. If the symptom worsens with increasing retractions and deteriorating blood gases increasing the level of CPAP may help, but sometimes the only option is to re-intubate the baby. Before the next extubation it is worth giving dexamethasone (0.5 mg/kg/day) to try and reduce laryngeal oedema.

Subglottic stenosis. This is usually only seen in the very small baby (<0.75 kg) following *very* prolonged intubation.

Surfactant replacement

Recently, numerous trials of treatment with various forms of artificial, synthetic and natural surfactant are currently being reported. All those which are properly carried out show some degree of benefit. Although this form of therapy is not yet in routine clinical practice, it is likely that it will become so within the next 5 years.

Prevention of RDS

Prevention of prematurity

Too little is yet known about the mechanisms that initiate premature labour and the aetiology of the complications that precipitate it to make this feasible. Drugs such as β stimulants are used to reduce uterine contractions and thus prevent labour from progressing; these may also stimulate the release of surfactant.

Corticosteroids

There is good experimental evidence that corticosteroids administered to the mother can accelerate lung maturation and thus enhance surfactant production. It is, however, notoriously difficult to assess the results of clinical trials because of the enormous number of variables (e.g. gestational age, birthweight, spontaneous labour, mode of delivery and complications). At present it seems that the only groups of infants likely to benefit are:
1 Female fetuses.
2 Those whose mothers have already started in labour which has been successfully delayed for at least 48 hours.
3 Gestational age 30–32 weeks.
4 Those without a contra-indication to steroid therapy, e.g. prolonged membrane rupture, pre-eclamptic toxaemia or diabetes mellitus.
Thus this represents a very small, highly-selected group who would be likely to do well with modern treatment in any case.

Intrapartum prevention

This really boils down to aiming to deliver a baby in the best possible condition; this is helped by:
1 Attention to maternal factors that might compromise the fetus, e.g. hypotension, blood gas disturbance.
2 *In utero* transfer of 'high risk' mothers, particularly if less than 30 weeks, to a centre with intensive care facilities.
3 Involving the paediatrician in decisions about delivery.
4 Adequate fetal monitoring.
5 Delivery by caesarean section if there is fetal distress before labour or in the first stage.
6 Elective caesarean section in breech presentations at 26–32 weeks.
7 Delivery and anaesthesia conducted by experienced staff.

Postpartum prevention

1 Swift, adequate resuscitation and good care in the first hour or two may make all the difference between a baby who gets either no respiratory distress or is only mildly affected, and one who has severe disease with all the potential for complications.
2 Early postnatal transfer to regional centres of babies under 32 weeks who manifest more than mild RDS.

Transient tachypnoea of the newborn (TTN)

This condition which usually affects term infants, but may also affect preterm ones causes respiratory distress starting shortly after birth. It is due to delayed clearance of lung liquid after birth and the infants often have mild surfactant abnormalities.

TTN has the following characteristics:
1 Intrauterine asphyxia is rare although the mother may have been heavily sedated.
2 It is commoner in infants born by caesarean section pre-labour.
3 The infant may be either tachypnoeic (100–120/minute without much grunting, or breathe at 40–60/minute and grunt loudly; thus this group merges into mild RDS (p.133). Retractions are not a prominent feature.
4 There may be cyanosis in air but hypoxia is readily relieved in 30–40% oxygen and there is no CO_2 retention.
5 Chest X-ray shows 'streaky' vascular markings extending from the hilum and fluid may be seen in the interlobar fissures.
6 Improvement is usually seen in 12–48 hours.
7 Survival is the rule.

Treatment

Give oxygen to control cyanosis but umbilical catheterization is needed only in preterm infants. Antibiotics (penicillin) are usually given until culture results are known (p.140). Intravenous fluids may be needed for a short time but oral feeds are tolerated within 24–48 hours.

Meconium aspiration

Aspiration of meconium into an infant's lungs can lead to serious problems at resuscitation (p.120) and subsequent severe pulmonary disease.

Pathogenesis

A mature fetus responds to intra-uterine hypoxia by passing meconium (premature fetuses virtually never do so). Meconium staining occurs in the liquor of 10–20% of births but most of these do not develop respiratory symptoms. In a few, large amounts are passed and the liquor resembles pea soup. If there is asphyxia and the baby gasps during labour or immediately after birth, some of this noxious material may be aspirated into the trachea and lungs. Plugging of the airways leads to air trapping and a consequent risk of pneumothorax (p.155). Meconium is also an irritant and leads to a chemical pneumonitis as well as providing a good culture medium for secondary bacterial infection.

Clinical features of the infants at risk

1 Mature or post mature.
2 Fetal distress in labour.
3 Skin, umbilical cord and nails may be deeply stained with meconium.
4 Thick meconium in oro-pharynx or trachea at birth.
For management at birth see p.119.

After resuscitation the infant develops all the signs of respiratory distress (p.127). In addition the chest appears over-inflated, and fine crepitations and ronchi are heard. Hypoxia may be profound. CO_2

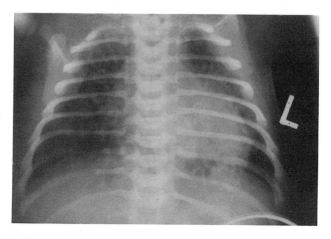

Fig. 15.7. Meconium aspiration.

retention is only seen when the condition is *very* severe; there may be a profound metabolic acidaemia due to the associated birth asphyxia. X-ray shows over-expansion and coarse infiltrates (Fig. 15.7). Ventilation is sometimes required and there is improvement in the clinical and radiological features over the next 7−14 days.

Complications

Plugging of the smaller airways leads to distal air trapping and a high risk of pneumothorax and pneumomediastinum. The asphyxia and hypoxia may cause secondary effects on:
1 Brain (cerebral oedema and convulsions).
2 Kidney (renal failure and acute tubular necrosis).
3 Myocardium (ischaemia and hypotension).

Management

1 Monitoring and intensive care along the same lines as that described for RDS are required (UAC, serial blood gases, etc., p.136).
2 Antibiotics, usually penicillin and gentamicin.
3 Oxygen. Give sufficient to keep the $P_a O_2 > 8$ kPa (60 mmHg); there is no risk of RLF in these infants. For persistent and severe hypoxia intravenous tolazoline may be useful (2 mg/kg stat, followed by infusion at 1 mg/kg/hour).
4 Hypercapnia. Always consider pneumothorax. Ventilation is needed if $P_a CO_2$ rises > 9.5 kPa (70 mmHg) particularly if $H^+ > 65$ nmol/l (pH < 7.2).
5 IPPV. Severe hypoxia ($P_a O_2 < 5$ kPa, 37.5 mmHg), particularly if combined with hypercapnia, is an indication for IPPV; these infants always need pancuronium (p.145).

Prognosis

The prognosis is good as far as the lungs are concerned. Long-term neurological outcome depends on the degree of asphyxia.

Pulmonary air leaks

This includes pneumothorax, pneumomediastinum, pneumopericardium, pneumoperitoneum, pulmonary interstitial emphysema, subcutaneous emphysema and systemic air embolism. These can be:

1 Spontaneous (pneumothorax, pneumomediastinum).
2 Secondary to barotrauma (all the above).

Mechanism

When alveolar rupture occurs, air tracks along the broncho-vascular bundles to the hilum where it dissects into the mediastinum and thence into the pleural space or pericardium, the subcutaneous tissues or into the peritoneum via the diaphragmatic foramina.

Pathogenesis of air leaks

1 The newborn infant exerts very high inspiratory pressures, particularly during the first few breaths (40–80 cmH_2O).
2 Plugging of the smaller airways, e.g. by meconium, leads to a ball valve effect with distal air trapping.
3 Barotrauma. Vigorous resuscitation or IPPV may cause alveolar rupture.

Pulmonary interstitial emphysema (PIE)

Multiple alveolar rupture with widespread dissection of air into the pulmonary interstitial space occurs predominantly in premature infants with RDS who are on IPPV. Diagnosis is by X-ray (Fig. 15.8), the lung fields resemble a snowstorm with multiple air-filled cysts contrasting with the collapsed and compressed lung tissue. The entrapped air severely interferes with blood gas exchange and frequently leads to a pneumothorax. It is of grave prognostic significance and is commonly the harbinger of BPD.

Management

Make every effort to minimize further barotrauma; keep inspiratory pressures to the minimum, fast ventilator rates at lower pressures may be successful; paralysis is usually indicated.

Pneumomediastinum

Most frequently seen in association with other air leaks but can occur in isolation and has the following features:
1 It can be completely asymptomatic and found by routine X-ray, or

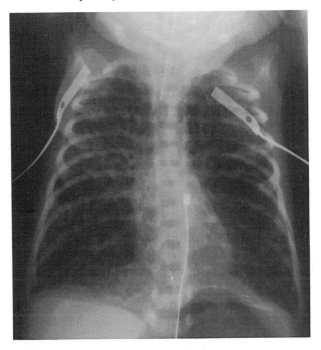

Fig. 15.8. Pulmonary interstitial emphysema. Note also the hyper-inflated lungs and the 'squashed' heart.

produce only minimal respiratory distress.

2 Tachypnoea and cyanosis may occur.

3 The anterior chest wall may be bowed forwards with a hyper-resonant percussion note.

4 There may be diminished air entry with distant heart sounds.

Diagnosis

Diagnosis is by X-ray which shows air in the mediastinum on frontal view; lateral view (horizontal beam, infant supine) shows air in the anterior mediastinum (Fig. 15.9).

Treatment

The mediastinal gas is loculated so that drainage is impracticable. In

(a)

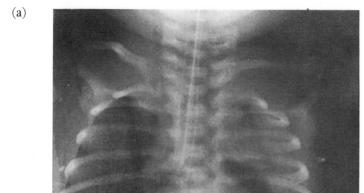

(b)

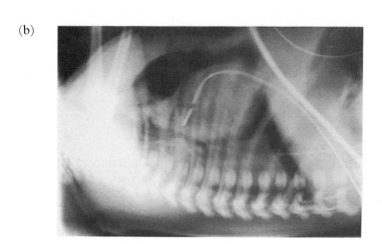

Fig. 15.9. Pneumomediastinum. (a) Anterior view. (b) Lateral view, note air in front of the heart.

mature infants resorption of air may be aided by giving high concentrations of oxygen; this replaces nitrogen and is then rapidly taken up by the circulation.

Pneumothorax

Small pneumothoraces may be asymptomatic and have been shown to occur in up to 1.5% of neonates. The incidence of pneumothorax in ventilated babies is about 30%. A large tension pneumothorax (Fig. 15.10) is one of the commonest neonatal emergencies and unless rapidly drained has grave consequences.

Infants at risk

1 Those with meconium aspiration.
2 All infants on CPAP or IPPV particularly if they are on peak pressures exceeding 25 cmH$_2$O and/or high mean airway pressures.
3 Those with PIE or pneumomediastinum.

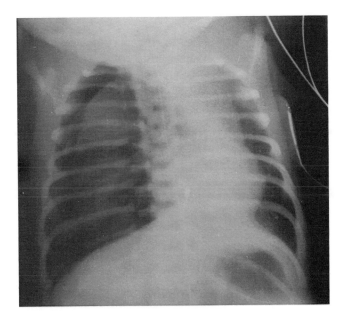

Fig. 15.10. A tension pneumothorax.

Clinical features

1 Sudden or gradual deterioration, e.g. increasing oxygen requirements, pallor, marked swings in BP.
2 Worsening blood gases. If there is hypoxia or a marked mediastinal shift compromising the venous return, a metabolic acidaemia may reflect the resulting hypoperfusion.
3 Clinical examination: bulging chest, hyper-resonant percussion note, diminished air entry on the affected side, abdominal distension. It is often difficult to elicit these signs in a baby on a ventilator with electrodes obscuring the chest and mechanical noises masking the sound.
4 Chest transillumination: this may show increased translucence on the affected side, but cannot be used to exclude the diagnosis.

Diagnosis is by X-ray. If the baby is *in extremis*, clinical suspicion is high or the radiographer is delayed, confirm the diagnosis by inserting a needle on a syringe with or without a 3-way tap into the second intercostal space in the mid-clavicular line and aspirating the air.

Immediate management

1 Insert an intercostal drain (FG 10 or 12) connected to an underwater seal and suction (10−15 cmH₂O).
2 Repeat the X-ray after drainage to check that the air has gone. If it has not, fiddle with the drain or insert a second one.

Subsequent management

1 Remember that the same thing can happen on the other side.
2 X-ray the chest at least once a day.
3 If the baby is on IPPV he usually needs paralysis; wait until the inspiratory pressures are low (<20 cmH₂O) before attempting to remove the drain.
4 When the drain has stopped bubbling for 24−48 hours, clamp it and X-ray after a few hours. If there is no reaccumulation of air, remove the drain and close the hole with Steristrips.

Complications of pneumothorax

1 Severe hypoxia and hypercapnia. This may not recover after drainage of the pneumothorax and much higher IPPV pressures may be needed to restore the blood gases to their previous levels.

2 The hypercapnia and hypoxia may predispose to PVH (p.215), particularly in VLBW infants.

3 Trauma to the lung during thoracentesis.

4 Extension of the air leak causing pneumopericardium, pneumoperitoneum, subcutaneous emphysema or air embolism.

5 Death.

Pulmonary haemorrhage

Isolated pulmonary haemorrhage is rare. It is usually associated with other conditions and is better described as haemorrhagic pulmonary oedema.

Conditions associated with pulmonary haemorrhage

- Severe birth asphyxia
- RDS especially if there is a PDA
- Infection
- Disseminated intravascular coagulation (DIC) or other generalized bleeding disorder
- Hypothermia
- Kernicterus
- Fluid overload
- Congestive heart failure from any cause including PDA

These conditions lead to left ventricular failure plus damage to the pulmonary capillaries so that fluid, followed by red blood cells, leaks into the alveoli. The diagnosis is obvious with bloody fluid emerging from the trachea sometimes in alarming quantities; the fluid has a haematocrit of 5−10%.

Management

1 Treat the underlying disorder.

2 IPPV with paralysis is always needed. Clinical and blood gas monitoring are the same as in RDS.

3 Pay careful attention to fluid balance; diuretics should be given.

4 Give antibiotics.

5 Transfuse if there is significant blood loss; but take care not to overload the circulation.

6 Treat any coagulopathy.

Chronic lung disease

With improved survival of the VLBW infant has come a spectrum of more chronic lung disease which often results in long-term oxygen dependency, a prolonged hospital stay and an increased susceptibility to lower respiratory tract infections in infancy. The exact pathogenesis of these conditions is poorly understood but the following should be considered:

1 The chronic effects of premature aeration on lungs that are structurally and functionally immature.
2 The sequelae of acute disease in the immature lung.
3 The effects of treatment of the acute disease.

The conditions considered here are bronchopulmonary dysplasia (BPD), chronic pulmonary insufficiency of prematurity (CPIP) and Wilson−Mikity syndrome (Table 15.2).

Broncho-pulmonary dysplasia

This is confined to infants who have been on IPPV.

Aetiological factors

1 Mechanical distortion of the airways and lung parenchyma during IPPV, particularly when high pressures are used or air leaks have occurred.
2 The presence of an endotracheal tube interfering with ciliary action and mucous clearance.
3 Infection with long-term IPPV.
4 Oxygen toxicity. This probably only plays a subsidiary role.
5 Pulmonary oedema due to fluid overload and/or a PDA.

Incidence

Rare in infants >1.5 kg. Probably 10−20% of infants <1.5 kg ventilated for RDS.

Clinical features

After the acute phase (IPPV + RDS) there is a prolonged period of oxygen dependency and CO_2 retention for which ventilation may or may not be needed. Tachypnoea and retractions persist.

Table 15.2. Features of chronic lung diseases in premature infants.

	Bronchopulmonary dysplasia	Chronic pulmonary insufficiency of prematurity	Wilson – Mikity syndrome
AETIOLOGY	Barotrauma during IPPV, fluid overload ? Reaction to ETT ? O_2 toxicity	? Chronic surfactant deficiency	Collapse of immature bronchi ? Recurrent episodes of inhalation
PATHOLOGY	Bronchial squamous metaplasia Obliterative bronchiolitis Interstitial fibrosis		Voluminous lungs Septal thickening Areas of over-expansion No fibrosis
INFANTS AFFECTED	Following IPPV for HMD	Normal at first or mild HMD	Normal at first, onset at 2–6 weeks
CLINICAL FEATURES	Hypoxia Hypercapnia Dyspnoea	Hypoxia Hypercapnia Recurrent apnoea	Hypoxia Hypercapnia Apnoea, dyspnoea
X-RAY APPEARANCES	Small cysts which enlarge, streaky intervening areas Hyperinflation	Hazy lung fields Small lung volume	Cysts and streaky infiltrates, upper lobe dominance. If severe and generalized looks similar to BPD
MANAGEMENT	Oxygen IPPV prn Treat PDA Diuretics Steroids	Oxygen Theophyline CPAP, IPPV prn	Oxygen CPAP, IPPV prn

Radiology

Initially small, cystic areas are scattered throughout the lungs which gradually enlarge to produce a hyperinflated appearance; there are intervening areas of streakiness representing peri-bronchial thickening and atelectasis (Fig. 15.11).

Management

1 Prevention, by trying to avoid:
   a High ventilator pressures and barotrauma.
   b Fluid overload.
2 Give sufficient oxygen to maintain P_aO_2, monitored by trans-

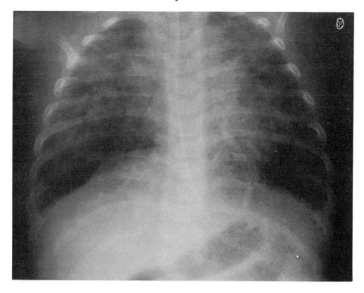

Fig. 15.11. Bronchopulmonary dysplasia.

cutaneous electrodes plus intermittent arterial blood sampling. Allow the P_aCO_2 to rise to $8-9$ kPa rather than reventilate or increase ventilator pressures.
3 Close a PDA if present.
4 Regular frusemide.
5 Dexamethasone seems to be beneficial.

Prognosis

Despite the need for 60% oxygen or more, sometimes for months, there are grounds for optimism in that there is great potential for continued alveolar development and regeneration. Every effort should be made to keep the P_aO_2 $>7-8$ kPa to prevent the development of permanent pulmonary hypertension. Good signs are coming off the ventilator, a gradual reduction in oxygen needs and a falling P_aCO_2. Ominous signs are rising ventilator requirements or reventilation, and the development of cor pulmonale.

Wilson Mikity syndrome

Clinical features

This rare condition occurs exclusively in premature infants who have either no RDS or only minimal symptoms over the first few days. They gradually develop dyspnoea and hypoxia after the first week or so, with increasing oxygen requirements over the next 2–6 weeks; CO_2 retention is usually mild. There is a tendency towards a slow recovery over several months.

Aetiology

Uncertain, but may be related to expiratory collapse of immature bronchi causing air trapping, or perhaps to the effects of the inhalation of small amounts of regurgitated milk.

Pathology

The lungs show areas of hyper-expansion, thickened septa and great variation in the size of the airspaces, particularly in the upper lobes (the usual site of aspiration in infants). Fibrosis is not prominent and the bronchial architecture is normal (cf. BPD).

Radiology

There is a cystic honeycomb appearance with intervening streaky areas most marked in the upper lobes.

Treatment

Give oxygen to relieve hypoxia but take care to avoid hyperoxia and the hazard of ROP.

Chronic pulmonary insufficiency of prematurity

This term is applied to a group of infants who manifest hypoxia and hypercapnia at a few weeks of age having been asymptomatic at first or having recovered from RDS. Clinically they are indistinguishable from the Wilson–Mikity group but radiologically the lungs are hazy and of small volume. Recovery over the next few weeks is the rule.

The cause has been ascribed to chronic (but transient) surfactant deficiency.

Treatment

Up to 40% oxygen may need to be given. Theophylline and CPAP may be useful.

Sequelae of lung disease in the neonate

Infants who have had RDS or one of the chronic lung diseases have an increased incidence of lower respiratory tract infections in infancy.

Recurrent apnoea

Most premature infants exhibit episodes of periodic breathing in which they are apnoeic for 5−10 seconds without any change in colour, then breathe at a rate of 50−60/minute. This phenomenon which occurs more often in REM sleep is about three times more common in infants <1.5 kg and gradually ceases by 34−36 weeks post conceptual age (Fig. 15.12).

Apnoeic attacks are usually defined as those in which the apnoea lasts for more than 20 seconds, often with bradycardia.

Aetiology

Symptomatic apnoea. This is a common and non-specific symptom of illness in ill, usually LBW infants.
Any of the following factors can act singly or alone:
1 Underlying lung disease, particularly if the infant becomes hypoxic.
2 Upper airway obstruction and mechanical interference. Obstruction of the nose by nasogastric tubes or secretions may induce reflex apnoea. Pharyngeal secretions or gastro-oesophageal reflex can interfere with breathing mechanically or in a reflex manner. Gastric distension by air or milk can compress the lung leading to hypoxia and apnoea.
3 Sepsis (p.172).
4 Heart failure (p.193).
5 Metabolic disturbance, e.g. hypoglycaemia (p.269), hypocalcaemia (p.236), hyponatraemia.
6 CNS disturbance, especially convulsions (p.208) and PVH (p.215).

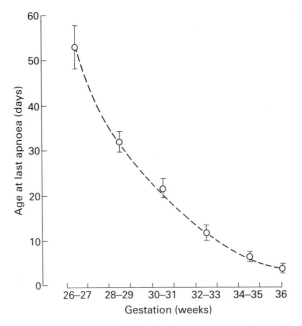

Fig. 15.12. Mean postnatal age ($\pm$S.E.) when last apnoea was detected vs gestational age at birth. (From Henderson-Smart *et al.*, 1978.)

7 Anaemia; infants with PCV <40%, particularly if unwell, are prone to apnoea.

Recurrent apnoea of prematurity

Many apparently normal preterm infants have recurrent apnoeic attacks for no obvious reason. They are thought to be due to 'immaturity' of the CNS control mechanism. The tendency to apnoea is inversely related to GA (Fig. 15.12).

Prevention of apnoea

Monitor all preterm infants at risk from apnoea so that attacks can be quickly recognized and dealt with; the methods used are:
1 A pressure sensitive capsule attached to the anterior abdominal wall which detects respiratory movements.
2 Lying the baby on a movement-sensitive mattress.
3 Attaching impedance electrodes to the baby's chest.
4 ECG monitoring which will detect bradycardia secondary to apnoea and hypoxia.

Avoid trigger factors such as hypoxia, bolus feeding of large quantities, hypoglycaemia, hypocalcaemia, anaemia.

Treatment of the acute apnoeic attack

Provided the apnoea is detected before marked hypoxia and bradycardia occur, the infant usually responds to simple stimulation. Attend to any other obvious precipitating cause such as secretions or a regurgitated feed. If apnoea persists resuscitate with a bag and mask using the same concentration of oxygen that the baby was having. Because these neonates are at major risk of ROP (p.317) only use pure oxygen for resuscitation if there is cyanosis and bradycardia unresponsive to the initial bag and mask resuscitation. Intubate if necessary.

Management and prevention of recurrent apnoea

1 Look for a cause (p.162) and treat it.
2 If the attacks are severe or the infant appears ill, start antibiotics after taking appropriate cultures (p.175).
3 If hypoxic (P_aO_2 <8 kPa [60 mmHg]), increase the F_IO_2 in steps of 2−5% with meticulous arterial or transcutaneous monitoring.
4 Oral theophylline (or intravenous aminophylline) is an effective respiratory stimulant.
5 Nasal prong CPAP is frequently helpful (p.32).
6 On rare occasions the only recourse is ventilation (IMV).

Prognosis

Provided any underlying condition can be adequately treated the outlook is excellent. There is no evidence that recurrent apnoea, *per se*, leads to brain damage.

Abnormalities of the larynx and trachea

Complete congenital obstructive lesions of the trachea and larynx are very rare and fatal.

Stridor

This is not an uncommon symptom in the neonate; it may be continuous or only heard during crying or be exacerbated during upper respiratory tract infections.

Aetiology and clinical features

1 Congenital stridor, laryngomalacia. The stridor sounds alarming but the infant is untroubled; it may begin in the neonatal period or be delayed several months. The stridor gradually lessens during infancy and disappears over the first year or two. The diagnosis is made by visualizing a large floppy epiglottis at laryngoscopy.

2 Intrinsic obstruction by webs, polyps or haemangiomata; these can all be seen at laryngoscopy.

3 Vocal cord paralysis unilateral or bilateral; visualized at laryngoscopy.

4 External compression by vascular rings, enlarged thyroid or cysts in the neck. These require contrast studies or CT scan to demonstrate them.

5 Laryngeal damage following prolonged endotracheal intubation, usually subglottic stenosis (p.147).

Management

1 All infants with persisting stridor should have a laryngoscopy. If this is normal consider further X-ray studies.

2 Do blood gases on infants with severe symptoms. Marked CO_2 retention indicates a need for further investigation and probably tracheostomy; This is a major undertaking in infants, not because it is particularly difficult but because it is extremely hard to decannulate infants, and the tube is likely to have to stay in for 2 or more years.

Congenital malformations of the respiratory tract

Upper airway obstruction

BILATERAL CHOANAL ATRESIA

This presents as marked respiratory distress at birth or immediately thereafter, because most infants are obligate nose breathers. The symptoms are intermittent and in contrast to most other forms of respiratory distress are relieved by crying. Diagnosis can be confirmed by:

1 Forcibly closing the mouth and observing deep retractions and prompt cyanosis.

2 Inability to pass a FG 5 suction catheter through either nostril.

3 In rare instances X-ray contrast studies are needed.

Treatment

1 Tape in an oral airway.

2 The definitive surgery consists of breaking through the posterior choanae and maintaining patency by inserting plastic tubes through both nostrils to the pharynx and leaving them in place until the passages have established themselves.

UNILATERAL CHOANAL ATRESIA

May not be diagnosed for weeks, months or even years. It may present as a unilateral purulent nasal discharge.

PIERRE ROBIN SYNDROME (mandibular hypoplasia, glossoptosis, cleft palate)

The basic defect is early (before 9 weeks fetal life) mandibular under-development so that the tongue is pushed backwards and impedes closure of the palate. The glossoptosis and micrognathia can lead to airway obstruction.

Clinical features

1 Small, receding jaw.
2 Rounded mid-line posterior cleft palate.
3 The tongue appears almost to fill the mouth.
4 Respiratory obstruction may be apparent at birth or may only become evident during feeding, and consists of retractions with or without cyanosis, choking, and stridor.

Management

There is an ever-present threat to the airway. Nurse the infant prone with the neck extended to try and prevent the glossoptosis. Nasopharyngeal CPAP may be of considerable value in infants with persisting airways problems. In an emergency use tongue forceps or a stitch through the tongue to pull it forwards. Intubation of these infants is extremely difficult and hazardous.

Prognosis

Mandibular growth and surgical closure of the palatal defect result in cure by 9–12 months of age. In the short-term if the airway obstruction is a persisting problem, tracheostomy will be needed.

Phrenic nerve palsy

This is very rare and is usually associated with an Erb's palsy (p.223).

Congenital abnormalities of the lungs

Agenesis

Agenesis of both lungs is extremely rare but unilateral agenesis does occur; there is compensatory hypertrophy of the contralateral lung, the infant may be asypmptomatic. Diagnosis is by X-ray.

Lung hypoplasia

Restriction of lung growth is usually secondary to some other factor:
1 Diaphragmatic hernia (p.244).
2 Fetal anuria resulting from lethal renal malformations (Potter's syndrome, p.283). The oligohydramnios leads to characteristic compression defects in the fetus which include 'Potter's' facies and pulmonary hypoplasia. The infant presents at birth as a resuscitation problem (p.122) and suffers severe respiratory distress. The condition is fatal.
3 Prolonged leak of amniotic fluid following ruptured membranes in the second trimester. The resulting oligohydramnios leads to compression defects which may be severe enough to cause pulmonary hypoplasia and 'Potter's' facies. If there is prolonged membrane rupture before 27 weeks the outlook may be bad, but if it occurs after this time the lungs are usually big enough to support life.

Antenatal diagnosis. In the presence of oligohydramnios without a demonstrable leak an attempt to establish a diagnosis should be made by searching for fetal kidneys and bladder with ultrasound. Visualization of a normal bladder and kidneys excludes Potter's syndrome. In such cases the fetus should be assumed to be normal.

Congenital lobar emphysema

In this uncommon condition there is over-distension of a single lobe with air-trapping and secondary compressive atelectasis of other areas. The affected lobe can herniate across to the opposite side with mediastinal shift leading to respiratory embarrassment. The upper lobes are most commonly affected, the left side more often than right.

Diagnosis. Symptoms can occur in the neonatal period or only arise during the first few months of life; they vary from mild wheezing to gross respiratory distress. Air entry is reduced over the affected area. X-ray reveals the overinflated lobe with partial or complete atelectasis of the other lobes and sometimes herniation with mediastinal shift.

Management. This depends on severity:
1 Mild symptoms call for supportive treatment and a 'wait and see' attitude because the emphysema may resolve spontaneously.
2 Occasionally lobectomy is indicated.

Congenital chylothorax/pleural effusion

The aetiology of this rare condition is unknown. More than half the infants become symptomatic within 24 hours of birth and present with non-specific signs of respiratory distress. X-ray reveals a pleural effusion. Thoracentesis yields clear fluid until after milk feeds have been introduced when it becomes frankly chylous. Males are twice as commonly affected as females. Treatment is by repeated thoracenteses and the use of an MCT milk.

Congenital adenomatoid malformation

This is a rare form of congenital cystic disease consisting of either multiple large cysts that resemble congenital lobar emphysema or much smaller cysts (<1.2 cm in diameter). Histology shows a polypoid proliferation of the respiratory epithelium. Clinically the infant presents with respiratory distress at or shortly after birth; half the cases are associated with hydrops. The only possible treatment is resection of the affected lobe.

Lymphangiectasia

Congenital dilatation of the lymphatic vessels may be confined to the lungs or associated with lymphangiectasia of other parts of the body. When confined to the lungs the condition usually occurs with congenital heart disease (particularly total anomalous pulmonary venous drainage). The true incidence is hard to determine. Infants who die with the condition show (in additon to the congenital heart disease) bulky lungs with pronounced lobulation, the septa are thickened due to the immensely dilated lymphatics.

References

Henderson Smart, D.J. (1978) The effect of gestational age on the incidence of recurrent apnoea. *Australian Paediatric Journal* 17, 273–76.

Roberton, N.R.C. (1986) *Manual of Neonatal Intensive Care*, 2nd edn. Edward Arnold and Co., London.

Further reading

Avery, M.E., Fletcher, B.D. & Williams, R.G. (1981) *The Lung and its Disorders in the Newborn Infant.* W.B. Saunders Co., Philadelphia.

Hodgman, J.E. (1981) Chronic Lung Disorders. In *Neonatology: Pathophysiology and Management of the Newborn*, G.B. Avery (ed.), J.B. Lippincott Co., Philadelphia. pp.398–411.

Morley, C.J. (1986) Respiratory distress syndrome. In *Textbook of Neonatology*, N.R.C. Roberton (ed.), Churchill Livingstone, Edinburgh.

Stahlman, M.T. (1981) Acute Respiratory Discorders in the Newborn. In *Neonatology: Pathophysiology and Management of the Newborn*, G.B. Avery (ed), J.B. Lippincott Co., Philadelphia, pp.371–97.

Thibeault, D.W. & Gregory, G.A. (1979) *Neonatal Respiratory Care.* Addison-Wesley, Menlo Park, California.

Vyas, H. & Milner, A.D. (1986) Other respiratory diseases in the neonate. In *Textbook of Neonatology*, N.R.C. Roberton (ed.), Churchill Livingstone, Edinburgh. pp.312–39.

Chapter 16
Infection in the Newborn

Host defences in the newborn

The body has three lines of defence against infection:
- Physical
- Cellular
- Humoral

All three are deficient in neonates.

Physical defences

These are the intact skin and mucous membranes, ciliary function and the presence of a normal bacterial flora. Neonatal skin is very thin and easily damaged and infected. The umbilical stump can become necrotic after birth and acts as a locus for infection (Chapter 9). The presence of an endotracheal tube or nasogastric tube or an intravascular catheter provides a route for pathogens to enter the body.

Humoral immunity

Normal neonates have no circulating IgA and IgM, but IgG is actively transported across the placenta from about the 20th week of gestation, so that by full term fetal IgG is higher than maternal. Following delivery the infant's IgG level falls until he starts to produce his own, so there is a transient postnatal hypogammaglobulinaemia. In term infants this is rarely important, but the premature infant, born before much IgG has crossed the placenta, not only starts life with a low IgG level, but develops marked postnatal hypogammaglobulinaemia with levels less than 10% of normal adult values.

Complement levels are 50–80% of adult values in the fullterm neonate, and even lower in premature infants.

Cellular immunity

The neonate has reduced lymphocyte and polymorphonuclear leucocyte function. The absolute number of T cells present is reduced by about 50%; the number of B cells is normal, but their ability to produce an antibody in response to antigen challenge is, however, reduced.

The low level of immunoglobulins and complement are primarily responsible for the poor chemotaxis and phagocytosis seen in neonates, since, when neonatal polymorphs are suspended in adult serum they perform normally. The ability of neonatal polymorphs to kill ingested pathogens, particularly coliforms, is reduced in the presence of serious illness such as RDS, meconium aspiration or septicaemia, and the neutrophil storage pool is rapidly depleted.

Effects of reduced host defences

The neonate is not only predisposed to infection, but when infection does occur it disseminates very rapidly and septicaemic shock and death can occur within 12 hours of the first signs of illness. This susceptibility, which is more marked the more immature the baby, has two major implications:

1 Early recognition of infectious disease is essential. Even trivial clinical findings suggesting infection demand meticulous evaluation.

2 Therapy must be started on the basis of clinical suspicion alone. There is no time to wait for bacteriology results to come back 24−48 hours later.

Bacterial infection in the newborn

The spectrum of bacteria which cause neonatal infection is different from that seen in older children and adults. *E. coli* and the group B β-haemolytic streptococcus (GBS) cause 70−85% of severe neonatal infection, and the organisms listed below are responsible for most of the other cases:

• Other streptococci (group A, D, G, *S. pneumoniae*, *S. viridans*, *S. faecalis*)
• *Staphylococcus aureus* and *S. epidermidis*
• Other gram negative bacilli (*Klebsiella, Proteus, Enterobacter*)
• *Pseudomonas aeruginosa*
• *Haemophilus* sp.
• *Listeria monocytogenes*
• *Serratia marcescens*
• Anaerobes

Superficial infections

Bacterial infection of the umbilicus and skin

This is often caused by *Staphylococcus aureus*, and to minimize it, the umbilical cord stump should be treated before the cord is clamped and daily thereafter with an antiseptic or antibiotic spray (Chapter 6). This usually prevents infection of the umbilicus, but if infection does break through, it usually responds rapidly to application of further topical antibiotics. The 'prophylactic' treatment of the cord from birth not only prevents portal pyaemia and systemic infection, but reduces the incidence of staphylococcal infections of the baby's skin and conjunctiva and the mother's breasts.

Nevertheless rare cases of staphylococcal skin infection with small superficial blisters are still seen, but respond rapidly to 5 days of oral flucloxacillin.

Thrush

This presents as white plaques on the buccal mucosa and tongue, or as a confluent perianal rash, with discrete peripheral lesions looking like the bases of small blisters. Thrush responds rapidly to topical nystatin.

Conjunctivitis

The diagnosis and management of this is outlined in Table 16.1.

Systemic bacterial infection

Detecting severe infection as early as possible is one of the major preoccupations of neonatal care. It depends initially on shrewd and vigilant nurses detecting the slight and subtle presentations of major infection particularly in the VLBW infant:

1 Listlessness, lethargy, hypotonia, pallor, mottled skin; the baby just does not seem right. These non-specific signs are often the first indication that a baby is infected.

2 Anorexia. If a previously healthy neonate refuses to feed, especially if this is because of dyspnoea, infection should be suspected.

3 Apnoea. Recurrent apnoeic attacks (p.162) are often the first sign of infection in premature infants.

4 Irritability. An irritable baby who won't stop crying or whimper-

Table 16.1. Treatment of neonatal conjunctivitis.

Organism	Age at presentation	Diagnosis	Treatment
Gonococcus	1 day (more cases now recognized later in first week)	Maternal history — promiscuity, etc. Profuse conjunctival discharge Urgent Gram stain on pus shows Gram −ve intracellular diplococci Culture of swab sent in transport medium	Intramuscular penicillin 75 000 units/kg/24 hours given bd Penicillin eye-drops hourly Notifiable disease Remember to treat mother and consorts
Staphylococcus aureus E. coli Haemophilus, pneumococcus, Streptococcus viridans	3−5 days peak, but may be at any time	Culture swab	If mild: sterile saline cleaning If severe: 0.5% chloramphenical drops for 5 days
Chlamydia trachomatis	7 days +	Venereal disease, therefore similar maternal history to gonococcus Conventional cultures sterile Chlamydial cultures positive Chlamydial immunofluorescence positive	Chlortetracycline eye ointment + systemic erythromycin (30 mg/kg) for at least 2 weeks

ing even for a feed may be developing a septicaemia or meningitis; alternatively it may indicate that he is in pain from bone or joint infection.

5 Pseudoparalysis. The lack of limb movement because of pain suggests arthritis or osteomyelitis.

6 Jaundice. If this develops rapidly in a neonate without haemolytic disease, sepsis is present until proved otherwise.

7 Vomiting. If persistent this is very suggestive of infection. Diarrhoea and vomiting are not necessarily signs of gastro-enteritis but are also common non-specific early features of infection.

8 Temperature change. Hypothermia and pyrexia are often due to defective environmental temperature control (p.41). However, a core temperature less than 36°C or more than 37.5°C sustained for more than an hour or two in the correct environmental temperature strongly suggests infection.

9 Tachypnoea. This is often the first sign of pneumonia or septicaemia.

10 Poor weight gain. This, without any other symptoms, can indicate occult infection though it is not a feature of acute infection.

11 System-specific signs of infection such as the following, are signs of well-established disease. If infection presents in these ways, the diagnosis could probably have been made earlier.

  a Pulmonary: cyanosis, grunting, respiratory distress and cough.

  b Abdominal: bilious or feculent vomiting, abdominal distension, livid flanks and periumbilical staining, absent bowel sounds and ileus.

  c Meningitis: a high-pitched cry, head retraction, bulging fontanelle and convulsions.

Clinical evaluation

1 Confirm the presenting history or symptoms.

2 Review the history:

  a Is the infant predisposed to infection in any way, e.g. very premature, arterial catheter, intubated?

  b Is there anything in the perinatal history increasing the likelihood of infection, e.g. maternal infection or pyrexia, prolonged rupture of membranes, pathogens in the mother's high vaginal swab?

  c Is the baby at risk from nosocomial infection from relatives, staff or other infants in the ward?

3 Completely undress and carefully examine the baby, paying particular attention to the following:

  a Are there any infected lesions of the skin or subcutaneous tissues?

Are there pits or skin defects over the spine to allow infection to enter?

b Is the infant dehydrated?

c Is there periodic breathing or tachypnoea?

d Are crepitations heard when listening to the chest?

e Is there hepatosplenomegaly, suggesting septicaemia or hepatitis?

f Is there kidney enlargement — a sign of septicaemia as well as urinary tract infection?

g Is the umbilicus red or tender with a thickened cord of inflamed umbilical vein extending up the falciform ligament?

h Can osteomyelitis and arthritis be excluded by demonstrating that limb movements are painless?

i Are bowel sounds present and is palpation of the abdomen painful, suggesting peritonitis?

j Is he tender in the renal angle — suggesting pyelonephritis?

4 Exclude otitis media.

Investigation

Whenever there is clinical suspicion of infection always carry out the following tests:

1 Swabs of nose, throat, umbilicus and any skin lesions. The swabs, if not plated immediately, should be put in transport medium.

2 Stool culture or effective rectal swabs.

3 Endotracheal tube aspirate (if relevant).

4 Bag urine. The vulva or penis should be cleaned as carefully as possible. Positive results from bag urine specimens in the neonate should always, however, be viewed with grave suspicion because of the great risk of contamination. If there is any doubt, collect urine by suprapubic bladder puncture (p.344).

5 Blood culture; this *must* be taken from direct arterial or venous puncture, and nowhere else.

6 WBC and a differential. After 48 hours of age, a polymorph count greater than $7.5-8 \times 10^9/l$ ($7500-8000/mm^3$) or less than $1-1.35 \times 10^9/l$ ($1000-1350/mm^3$), $> 0.8 \times 10^9/l$ ($800/mm^3$) myelocytes, and a left shift or toxic granulation of the white cells are all very suggestive of bacterial infection. On day 1, a total white count less than $6.5 \times 10^9/l$ ($6500/mm^3$) or less than $2.5 \times 10^9/l$ ($2500/mm^3$) polymorphs also suggest infection.

7 Chest X-ray.

8 In the case of infants who develop symptoms within a few hours of delivery, in addition to the above tests, Gram stain and culture the gastric aspirate and swabs from the external auditory meatus, and arrange for a maternal high vaginal swab to be taken.

The following procedures should be carried out in most instances but some discretion can be applied before doing them on all infants with the merest suggestion of infection:

1 Lumbar puncture. This should usually be carried out unless there is a clear-cut primary focus of infection such as pneumonia in an infant on a ventilator.

2 Abdominal X-ray; always do one if there is abdominal distension or rectal bleeding.

3 Blood gases: a metabolic acidaemia often occurs in severe infection: if the base deficit is >10 mmol/l not only does it suggest sepsis, but it should be corrected.

Treatment of infection

Antibiotics

The most difficult part of antibiotic therapy is deciding when to start it. However, since it is usually impossible to exclude infection as the cause of the abnormal clinical and laboratory findings, most neonates suspected of infection should be given antibiotics. These can be stopped in 5 days or less if the patient rapidly improves, and the cultures are negative. Proven localized infections such as pneumonia or a urinary tract infection should have at least 10 days' treatment, rising to at least 14 days in septicaemia. Antibiotics should be given i.v., since i.m. antibiotics in the neonate may damage nerve and muscle, and it is doubtful if oral antibiotics have any role in serious systemic neonatal infection.

Two antibiotics should always be given. To treat coliform infection one of these should be an aminoglycoside such as gentamicin. Depending on which of the following organisms are common in the unit select the second, or even third antibiotic from:

• Penicillin G for group B haemolytic streptococci
• Flucloxacillin for *Staphylococcus (S.epidermidis or S.aureus)*
• Ceftazidime or piperacillin for *Pseudomonas aeruginosa*
• Ampicillin for *Listeria monocytogenes*

In patients with NEC give metronidazole to deal with anaerobes.

Acid base data/blood gases

Septicaemic infants are often acidaemic and hypoxic. The indications for, and management of, intravenous base, supplementary oxygen and IPPV are identical to those in RDS (p.136 *et seq.*).

Hypotension

This is common in septicaemic infants and should be treated initially with plasma or blood transfusions. Intravenous dopamine should be tried if hypotension (<35 mmHg systolic) persists.

Haemostasis

DIC (p.291) may occur in severe septicaemia, and should be treated with fresh frozen plasma or blood transfusion. Heparinization is not indicated.

Exchange transfusion

As well as being good for DIC and hypotension, fresh blood contains the immunoglobulins and opsonins, the lack of which predisposes infants to septicaemia. Exchange transfusion has been shown to improve the prognosis in severe septicaemia, particularly if sclerema (p.182) is developing.

Specific bacterial infections in the neonate

Early onset septicaemia and pneumonia (GBS septicaemia)

During the last 10 years it has been recognized that many infants of all gestations who die in the first 24 hours of life have an overwhelming septicaemia. The infecting organisms are acquired intrapartum from the mother's birth canal, where they are usually commensals. The commonest cause in the group B β-haemolytic streptococcus (GBS) but most of the organisms listed on p.171 can be responsible. In a typical case of GBS septicaemia at term, the infant, who was a normal delivery without prolonged rupture of the membranes or asphyxia develops mild grunting and recession and needs 30–40% oxygen aged 1–2 hours, but he is vigorous, and does not appear to be critically ill.

Aged 6–8 hours he collapses with peripheral vasoconstriction, severe hypoxia and acidaemia. The chest X-ray shows bilateral patchy changes suggesting pneumonia. Despite antibiotics, IPPV, high oxygen concentrations and infusions of base, the clinical abnormalities persist and the infant dies, aged on average 14–16 hours.

In preterm infants the presentation is with respiratory distress (p.134), but instead of showing a sustained improvement when ventilated within the first few hours, the baby becomes progressively more hypoxic, acidaemic and hypotensive with, like his fullterm counterpart, a fatal outcome.

To prevent this type of disaster, after taking appropriate cultures (see above):

1 Give a single dose of i.m. benzylpenicillin 50 000/kg to all asymptomatic infants delivered to mothers known to be carrying GBS.

2 Give i.v. benzylpenicillin to any neonate who shows any signs of respiratory illness within a few hours of delivery, and keep him on this until the cultures are known to be negative for GBS. If GBS is grown, or if other suspicious features are present (p.174) the dose of benzylpenicillin should be doubled and gentamicin added.

Pneumonia

This is caused by any of the organisms responsible for neonatal septicaemia (p.171). Viral pneumonia is rare in the neonate. Respiratory illness coming on after 4 hours (p.127) of age in an infant who does not have heart failure, or a pneumothorax or lung malformation on a chest X-ray, is due to pneumonia until proved otherwise. Infants with pneumonia may have abnormal physical signs on chest auscultation, but usually the only abnormal signs are those of respiratory distress. The chest X-ray may show patchy consolidation which is diagnostic, but commonly all that is seen is some non-specific haziness.

If pneumonia develops in the first 24 hours, GBS infection is likely, and, after taking the appropriate cultures (p.175) and checking the blood count, penicillin and gentamicin should be given intravenously. After 48 hours of age, staphylococcal disease is more likely and flucloxacillin should be added to the gentamicin.

Pneumonia in the infant on IPPV

The presence of an endotracheal tube for more than 24−48 hours considerably increases the risk of pneumonia. Should the clinical condition of an infant, ventilated for any reason, begin to deteriorate, pneumonia must always be considered. This diagnosis is more likely if:

- The secretions up the endotracheal tube are purulent
- The baby shows other 'non-specific' signs of infection (p.173)

- The baby is febrile
- There is a neutrophil leucocytosis
- There is new patchy consolidation on the CXR

Appropriate investigations including blood culture and culture of the endotracheal tube aspirate should always be done, but if the clinical suspicion of infection is strong enough, appropriate antibiotics (see above) should be started at once.

Neonatal meningitis

The traditional signs of a bulging fontanelle, head retraction, and a high-pitched cry are those of established meningitis which has progressed to a cerebritis and cortical thrombophlebitis. The mortality and long-term neurological morbidity of such infants is high, and every effort should be made to diagnose neonatal meningitis when the signs are minimal (p.174).

Diagnosis

The diagnosis of meningitis is based on examination of the cerebrospinal fluid (CSF), by cell count, culture and biochemical analysis. The following suggest meningitis:

1 A CSF polymorph count greater than 20/mm^3.
2 Organisms seen on Gram stain and grown on culture.
3 Positive tests for bacterial antigens, e.g. latex agglutination tests.
4 CSF glucose less than 1 mmol/l or much lower than a simultaneous blood glucose. The CSF protein is rarely helpful.

Treatment

Neonatal meningitis is a major emergency, and should only be managed in a centre with full microbiological, neurosurgical and neuroradiological facilities.

The basic treatment is that described for septicaemia described above. However, the antibiotics used and their route of administration have to be chosen not only on the basis of the likely sensitivities of the organisms seen on the Gram stain of the CSF, but also on the basis of whether or not they penetrate the CSF. The availability of the newer broad spectrum, third generation cephalosporins which penetrate well into the CSF has revolutionized the treatment of neonatal meningitis, and means that intrathecal therapy, and in particular intraventricular therapy, are now rarely needed.

The three organisms most commonly responsible for neonatal meningitis are group B streptococci, *E. coli* and *Listeria*. The appropriate antibiotic combination given intravenously for these is:
- Group B streptococci — penicillin and gentamicin
- *Listeria* — ampicillin and gentamicin
- *E. coli* — ceftazidime or cefotaxime plus gentamicin

For other organisms the appropriate antibiotics should be chosen in consultation with the local bacteriologist.

The infant should have lumbar punctures daily for the first few days, and it is essential to measure regularly the antibiotic levels in plasma and CSF to ensure that adequate doses have been given. If the infection is not clearing, then consideration should be given to intrathecal therapy. Using the antibiotic cocktails outlined above this is only likely to be a problem with coliform meningitis or meningitis due to the other rare Gram-negative bacilli. In these babies a ventriculitis is almost certain to be present. This should be confirmed by ventricular puncture followed by intraventricular antibiotics. If these are needed for more than 2−3 days an indwelling ventricular cannula and reservoir (Ommaya, Rickham) should be inserted.

Once the CSF cell count and protein levels are falling, and the CSF becomes sterile, the frequency of lumbar punctures can decrease, but one should always be done before stopping therapy, and a final one 2−3 days later. Antibiotics should be given i.v. to infants with neonatal meningitis for at least 3 weeks.

Complications

Common complications in infants with meningitis are listed below with the appropriate therapy:

Complications	Treatment
Fits	Anticonvulsants
Cerebral oedema	Diuretics and mannitol
Inappropriate ADH production	Fluid restriction
Intestinal stasis and ileus	Intravenous feeding
Hydrocephalus	Shunting

Sequelae

The mortality from neonatal meningitis is 10−20%, with 10−30%

of survivors having serious neurological sequelae, including hydrocephalus, mental defect, cerebral palsy and deafness.

Urinary tract infection (UTI)

This often presents with mild symptoms — vomiting, poor weight gain, persisting anaemia or mild jaundice, though sometimes all the signs of severe sepsis are present. Care should be taken in diagnosing UTI on the basis of bag urine analysis. If a bag urine is normal, then the infant does not have a urinary tract infection. Bag urines with less than 50 cells/mm^3 without bacterial growth, or urines with a significant bacterial growth ($>10^5$ organisms/ml) without pyuria, should not be treated as a UTI without confirmation in urine obtained by suprapubic bladder puncture. However, a bag urine with a pure growth of $>10^5$ organisms/ml, plus $>100-200$ WBC/mm^3, is adequate proof of a UTI, provided that there was no local genital infection when the bag sample was collected. In infants with mild symptoms oral antibiotics such as amoxycillin can be given, but if the infant is more seriously ill i.v. gentamicin should be given for 10 days.

All neonates with a UTI should have their blood urea and electrolytes checked, and the process should be repeated following completion of therapy. Renal ultrasound, an appropriate radionuclide scan (DTPA or hippuran) and a micturating cystogram must also be carried out as quickly as possible to exclude congenital abnormalities.

Gastro-enteritis

Cases of gastro-enteritis in the neonatal period are usually sporadic, but occasional outbreaks still occur, mainly due to rotavirus or enteropathogenic *E. coli*.

Diagnosis

This is obvious in the infant with vomiting and frequent loose, watery stools. These stools should be cultured, and, if indicated, checked for viruses by electron microscopy.

Treatment

In mild gastro-enteritis, stop milk feeds and give one of the commercial glucose electrolyte solutions such as Dioralyte or Dextrolyte. In most cases the diarrhoea will settle within 24 hours, and milk-feeding can restart. If the diarrhoea does not settle, or dehydration develops, intravenous therapy will be required for 24–48 hours before restarting oral fluids.

If a term infant develops gastro-enteritis on the PNW do not admit him to the NNU. If he can be managed on oral treatment, transfer him and his mother to the maternity isolation ward. If he requires intravenous therapy he should be transferred to the hospital infectious disease unit if possible with his mother. If the infant is already on the NNU, keep him there, but institute full barrier nursing.

One point to remember about gastro-enteritis in the newborn is that severe diarrhoea without vomiting which responds to clear fluid but relapses when milk is introduced suggests congenital sugar intolerance (p.252).

Sclerema

This condition, which occurs in newborn infants, is a form of firm subcutaneous oedema with sluggish capillary perfusion and a waxy appearing skin. It is often found in infants with a severe infection, but may also occur in other very sick babies.

In the past most cases died. Recently, considerable success has been reported from exchange transfusion in infected infants with sclerema.

Virus infections

Viruses may cause severe neonatal infection. The signs, symptoms and investigations are identical to those seen in bacterial infections, and the management is exactly the same, including the use of exchange tranfusion. Antibiotics are given initially for the usual reasons in a clinically seriously ill septic infant, but they can be stopped once the viral aetiology is established. Any infant with clinical evidence of overwhelming sepsis from whom no bacteria are cultured after 48 hours' incubation should be suspected of a viral infection. Samples of stool, CSF and naso-pharyngeal aspirate in appropriate virus transport medium should be sent for viral culture. Viral culture should also be done at post-mortem in all unexplained 'septicaemic' neonatal deaths.

Coxsackie group B myocarditis

This presents at 5–10 days with fever, listlessness, tachycardia, tachypnoea, cyanosis, mottling and poor peripheral circulation. The infant is in heart failure and is usually hypotensive. Chest X-ray shows cardiomegaly, and the ECG shows changes of cardiomyopathy. There may be a coexisting viral meningitis.

Treatment

Digitalize the infant (with great care) and give diuretics; support the neonate with all the techniques of intensive care. In some instances, this will tide him over the acute illness, but the majority die.

Enteroviral infections

These may cause severe and often fatal infections characterized by all the signs of severe septicaemia outlined above — hypotension, jaundice, DIC and temperature instability: abdominal distension and tenderness are often seen. Echo 11 has commonly been isolated, but other echoviruses may be responsible. The diagnosis is made from cultures of CSF or stool.

As well as the standard therapy for major neonatal infection (p.176) the babies may benefit from injections of pooled human immunoglobulin. This may also be given to contacts to minimize the risk of nosocomial spread.

Viral respiratory infections

VLBW infants who stay in an NNU for several months, particularly if they have bronchopulmonary dysplasia (BPD) are very prone to develop severe illness if they contact the common respiratory viral infections to which 3−4 month-old infants are susceptible. Infection with respiratory syncytial virus (bronchiolitis) in such infants can be devastating, often causing respiratory failure needing 2−3 weeks of IPPV.

Neonatal herpes

The neonate may be infected by being delivered through a birth canal infected with type II (genital) herpes. For this reason, in the presence of overt genital herpes, infants should be delivered by caesarean section. However, most cases arise in neonates delivered from an apparently uninfected mother.

In its mildest form, neonatal herpes presents as a vesicular rash, but in the disseminated form, all the signs of severe neonatal sepsis are present, with jaundice, bleeding and cardio-respiratory collapse, plus

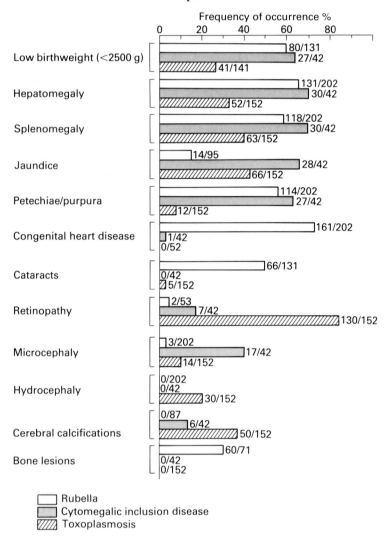

Fig. 16.1. Incidence of various defects in congenitally infected neonates. (From Overall & Glasgow, 1970.)

the more specific signs of keratitis, chorioretinitis and encephalitis.

The diagnosis can be made by electron microscopy of the vesicle fluid, or by culture of the virus from the vesicles, urine, eye lesions or the CSF.

Infants with neonatal herpes should be treated with intravenous acyclovir, though the morbidity and mortality remains high.

Congenital infections

The most common congenital infection (approx. 1:200 of all live births) is cytomegalovirus (CMV), which is usually asymptomatic in the neonatal period, although the infant may have a small head and be deaf on follow-up.

The other congenital infections, rubella, herpes virus (very rare) and toxoplasma, in addition to CMV may present in the neonatal period with the following conditions (Fig. 16.1):

- Low birthweight for gestational age
- Jaundice
- Hepatosplenomegaly
- Thrombocytopenia and purpura
- Cataract
- Chorioretinitis
- Abnormalities of head growth/intracranial calcification
- Osteitis
- Congenital heart disease

Diagnosis

If these features are present, culture throat swabs, urine and CSF for viruses, and test the infant's blood for the presence of IgM specific for the organism in question. There is no treatment for congenital herpes, CMV or rubella, but congenital toxoplasmosis responds to spiramycin alternating with pyrimethamine plus sulphadiazine.

Congenital syphilis

This is now rare. If it is diagnosed on the basis of a SFD neonate with a bloody nasal discharge, jaundice, hepatomegaly and rash, and a mother with an appropriate history, the diagnosis can be confirmed by dark ground illumination of the nasal discharge or the content of skin bullae and vesicles. The infant will also have a positive serological test for syphilis in his IgM fraction.

A lumbar puncture should always be carried out to exclude CNS involvement.

Treat with procaine penicillin 50 000/kg daily for 2 weeks. This treats the congenital neurosyphilis as well. Do not forget to treat the mother — and her consorts!

Reference

Overall, J.C. Glasgow, L.A. (1970) Virus infections of the fetus and newborn infant. *Journal of Pediatrics* 77, 315–33.

Further reading

Davies, P.A. & Gothefors, L. (1984) *Bacterial Infections of the Fetus and Newborn Infant.* W.B. Saunders Co., Philadelphia.

Pearse, R.G. & Roberton, N.R.C. (1986) Infection in the newborn. In *Textbook of Neonatology*, N.R.C. Roberton (ed.), Churchill Livingstone, Edinburgh. p.725.

Remington, J.S. & Klein, J.O. (eds.) (1983) *Infectious Disease of the Fetus and Newborn Infant*, W.B. Saunders Co., Philadelphia.

Chapter 17
Cardiac Problems in the Newborn

Incidence

Congenital heart disease (CHD) has an incidence of about 7−8:1000 LB, and about 0.7:1000 LB have non-structural heart disease.

The types of CHD which cause problems in the neonatal period are different from the incidence of the different types of CHD in the whole population (Table 17.1). About a quarter of all infants with CHD require urgent assessment and therapy in the neonatal period, and despite the many recent advances in surgical technology, 20−25% of these die. Lethal CHD therefore contributes about 0.5−1/1000 to the current overall neonatal mortality of 5.5/1000 LB.

Assessment

Cardiac problems present in one of four ways in the neonatal period:
1 The asymptomatic infant with a murmur. Most infants with murmurs on day 1 do not have CHD.

Table 17.1. Incidence of heart malformation (after Rowe *et al.*, 1981).

	Incidence at all ages (%)	Incidence in neonatal period (%)
VSD	28	13
ASD	10	—
Pulmonary stenosis	10	3
Patent ductus	10	30
Tetralogy of Fallot	10	4
Aortic stenosis	7	—
Coarctation of aorta	5	7
Transposition of the great vessels	5	12
Hypoplastic left heart	—	9
Other	15	22
	100	100

2 Heart failure.
3 Cyanosis.
4 The presence of an arrhythmia.
In all four situations the evaluation of the neonate should proceed along identical lines, but clearly an ill infant will need more extensive investigation than one who is asymptomatic.

History

1 Is there a family history of CHD?
2 Was the mother ill during pregnancy, e.g. rubella, systemic lupus (p.207)?
3 Did the mother take any drugs during pregnancy, e.g. phenytoin, lithium?
4 Has the baby any signs noted by the nurses or the mother suggesting heart disease, such as breathlessness particularly with feeding, reluctance to feed, sweating, pallor, mottling, lassitude or cyanosis? These features are usually only present in an ill infant; in the majority of neonates with murmurs, they will be absent.
5 Has the baby been ill in any other way that might predispose to heart disease, e.g. infection (myocarditis), asphyxia (myocardial ischaemia) fluid-overload (congestive heart failure)?

Examination

This is outlined in full in Chapter 7.

Murmurs

Remember that a murmur is noted in 75% of normal neonates in the first 24 hours. The majority of these infants do not have significant CHD (see below); conversely, serious and potentially fatal heart disease may exist without any murmurs being detected in the first 24—48 hours.

Investigation

An ECG and chest X-ray is required in infants thought to have a 'significant murmur' (see below). In addition the following tests may be indicated, either to differentiate extra-cardiac causes of heart failure from CHD, or to evaluate the severity of illness in an infant with heart failure:
• Full blood count

- Urea and electrolytes
- Calcium and glucose
- Infection screen
- Blood gases

Chest X-ray (CXR)

A cardio-thoracic ratio of over 60% is above the normal limit in the neonate. The aortic arch is usually on the left, but may be right-sided in infants with tetralogy of Fallot, truncus arteriosus, and occasionally in rarer lesions. In left-sided heart failure the pulmonary arteries dilate, their margins become fuzzy and there is generalized lung haziness due to interstitial and alveolar oedema; there may be fluid in the right interlobar fissure, or even small pleural effusions.

If the CXR shows dextrocardia, check the position of the abdominal viscera. If the viscera are the mirror image of normal (liver on left, stomach on right) dextrocardia is not associated with CHD. In all other situations it is.

Electrocardiogram (ECG)

There are only minor differences between the ECG of the term and preterm infant. The values for normal amplitude of the QRS complex, the normal RS ratio and the normal QRS axis are given in the Appendix (Table A6).

To work out the QRS axis consider leads 1 and aVF, and find the net amplitude of these two leads by subtracting the negative deflection from the positive deflection. These values can then be plotted on a graph as in Fig. 17.1. The mean neonatal QRS axis is $+135°$ with a normal range of $+110$ to $+180$.

Signs of right ventricular hypertrophy

1 qR in V_1.
2 R in aVR, V_1, or V_2 greater than the upper limit of normal (Appendix, Table A6).
3 S in V_5 and V_6 greater than the upper limit of normal.
4 T in V_1 positive after day 3, provided it is also upright in V_5 and V_6.
5 R/S ratio in V_1 and V_2 greater than upper limit of normal (Appendix, Table A6).
6 Right axis deviation greater than $+180°$.

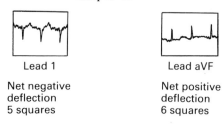

Lead 1   Lead aVF

Net negative   Net positive
deflection   deflection
5 squares   6 squares

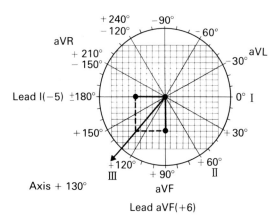

Axis + 130°

Lead aVF(+6)

Fig. 17.1. Diagram for working out QRS axis. Net deflections of each standard lead are plotted on the grid on the axes marked I, II, III, aVR, aVL and aVF. In practice all that is usually necessary is to plot lead I and lead aVF.

Signs of left ventricular hypertrophy

1 S in V_1 or V_2 greater than upper limit of normal.
2 R in I, II, III, aVL, aVF, V_5 or V_6 greater than the upper limit of normal.
3 R/S in V_1 less than lower limit of normal.
4 QRS axis of less than +30.
5 Q in V_5 and V_6 above upper limit of normal.

Signs of combined ventricular hypertrophy

1 Direct signs of 1 and 2.
2 Signs of 1, plus:
  a q of 2 mm or more over the left chest leads.
  b T inversion over the left chest leads after 3 days (with positive T in right chest leads).

3 Signs of 2, plus sizeable R or R' in the right precordial leads.
4 Mid-precordial leads of R + S more than 60 mm (Katz-Wachtel phenomenon).

Echocardiography

The continuing rapid developments in ultrasonic diagnostic equipment have revolutionized the investigation of neonatal CHD. Using two-dimensional echocardiography, it is now possible to get a clear picture of the internal anatomy of the heart painlessly and non-invasively.

In most infants in whom it is necessary to establish the nature of the defect responsible for heart failure or cyanosis, it is now possible to make an anatomical diagnosis by echocardiography alone. If cardiac catherization or angiocardiography are still necessary, these investigations can be planned in the light of the echocardiographic findings.

The infant with an asymptomatic murmur

Careful auscultation of the heart under ideal conditions will detect a systolic murmur in the first 48 hours of life in up to 75% of apparently healthy fullterm infants, yet less than 1% of them will turn out to have CHD. In most cases the murmur is soft, grade 1−2/6 and/or early systolic, but in about 10%, the murmur, although of similar intensity, is pansystolic. It is often possible to separate the 'significant' murmurs from the 'non-significant' ones on the basis of:
1 Loudness and duration: significant murmurs are likely to be louder, occupy more of systole or to have a coexisting thrill.
2 Other abnormalities on auscultation: abnormal second sound, triple rhythm, diastolic murmur.
3 The absence of femoral pulses.
4 Cyanosis.
However, even after examination by an experienced cardiologist only 15−20% of those thought to have a 'significant' murmur turn out to have CHD. In the remaining 80−85% the murmur will disappear, probably because it was due to:
● Transient patency of the ductus arteriosus
● Turbulence at the bifurcation of the pulmonary artery
● A small VSD, which subsequently closes
    In an infant with a murmur in the first 72 hours of life, in the absence of heart failure or any of the extra 'significant' auscultatory

findings, it is legitimate to hold a watching brief. However, if the murmur is thought to be significant the baby should have a CXR and ECG. If these are abnormal, early assessment by echocardiography is indicated. The conditions most likely to present in this way are ventricular septal defect (VSD), coarctation, a patent ductus, and various complex defects.

If the CXR and ECG are normal, the baby can be discharged from the hospital, but needs follow-up. In many, the murmur will disappear. In those in whom it does not, the likely diagnoses are:
- VSD
- PS
- AS
- Tetralogy of Fallot
- PDA

The distinctive auscultatory, radiological and ECG features of these conditions will become more apparent in the following months when the diagnoses should be confirmed echocardiographically.

Heart failure in the neonate

Clinical features

1 Pallor, lassitude, mottling, sweating, poor feeding.
2 Increased heart rate — always suspect heart failure if the pulse rate is greater than 160/minute in a term infant, or greater than 180/minute in a preterm infant.
3 A triple rhythm.
4 Increased respiratory rate in the absence of primary pulmonary disease. A respiratory rate >60/minute, with dyspnoea, suggests left ventricular failure with pulmonary oedema.
5 Crepitations heard in the lungs.
6 Apnoeic episodes ± bradycardia (especially in preterm infants).
7 Hepato-splenomegaly or a raised JVP.
8 Peripheral oedema is a rare and late feature in infants with congestive heart failure. However, a weight gain of more than 30 g/day suggests the fluid retention of heart failure.
9 Cardiomegaly — this is difficult to assess clinically in the neonate, but if noted radiologically it is strong evidence for heart failure.

Causes of heart failure in the neonate

This can be caused by non-structural heart disease (p.199). More commonly, heart failure is due to a structural congenital heart defect, and is best classified in a physiological way:

1 Structural defects with the systemic supply dependent on a patent ductus, e.g. interrupted aortic arch, hypoplastic left heart.
2 Severe left heart obstruction, e.g. severe congenital mitral or aortic stenosis, coarctation.
3 Valvular regurgitation, e.g. atrio-ventricular canal.
4 Left-to-right shunt *plus* another problem such as hypoxaemia (transposition + large VSD) valvular regurgitation (truncus) or immature myocardium (PDA in preterm infants).

Since the duct usually closes within 48−72 hours of delivery, conditions in group 1 will present at that time. However, conditions in groups 2−4 can present at any time during the first 1−2 months, with more severe examples presenting earlier. Heart failure due to isolated left to right shunts, e.g. PDA, VSD rarely presents in term babies until some weeks beyond the neonatal period.

Patent ductus arteriosus (PDA)

Aetiology

The incidence of PDA (Table 17.1) is particularly high in VLBW infants. In infants less than 1.5 kg, who require IPPV for RDS (p.139), the incidence may reach 50%. The reasons for this include:
1 Decreased sensitivity of the neonatal ductus to the oxygen stimulus to closure.
2 In the presence of severe lung disease recurrent episodes of hypoxia opening up the duct.
3 High circulating levels of PGE (a powerful ductus dilator).
4 Excess intravenous fluid therapy (Chapter 19).

Symptoms and signs

In both term and preterm infants PDA may present with just a murmur or the signs of heart failure, but by far the commonest situation is the appearance of a murmur in a preterm infant recovering, on IPPV, from severe RDS. The murmur is harsh, and audible at the left upper sternal border; it may extend into early diastole. The baby has a tachycardia, with bounding pulses; his heart sounds are normal, though there is often a gallop rhythm. His inspired oxygen requirement increases, his P_aCO_2 rises, and he needs more vigorous IPPV to keep his blood gases normal.

In term infants with a patent ductus a continuous murmur is common. Term infants should always be checked for signs of rubella syndrome.

CXR: Increased heart size and pulmonary plethora.

ECG: Often unhelpful, but with large shunts signs of ventricular overload may be seen.

Diagnosis

This is confirmed by demonstrating the patent ductus echocardiographically.

Treatment

Control the heart failure (p.198). Increase the ventilator settings if necessary. In the preterm infant, give oral or i.v. indomethacin (0.1–0.2 mg kg/8-hourly). This closes the ductus in about 75% of cases and can be repeated if necessary. It is less effective in the very premature (<30 weeks), the mature (>35 weeks), and those who, irrespective of gestation, are more than 3 weeks old. Ligation is necessary if, despite indomethacin, symptoms persist.

VSD

Although cases of VSD (Table 17.1) may present during the first week with a systolic murmur, symptoms are unlikely at this stage unless another lesion is present such as coarctation or PDA. Even infants with large VSDs will not develop signs of heart failure until 10–12 weeks of age when the postnatal fall in pulmonary artery pressure, and thus right ventricular pressure, allows a large left-to-right shunt to occur through the defect.

Symptoms and signs

The first heart sound is normal, but P_2 may be loud. There is a harsh pan-systolic murmur often with a thrill, and there may be a mid-diastolic murmur due to the large left-to-right shunt and consequent torrential flow across the mitral valve. Signs of heart failure may be present.

CXR: Except for very small defects, cardiomegaly with pulmonary plethora.

ECG: Small defects may have normal traces, or slight ventricular hypertrophy; with large defects a combined ventricular hypertrophy and overload patterns are seen.

Diagnosis

This can be confirmed, and the defect measured by echocardiography.

Treatment

The baby should be treated for heart failure, but if he does not respond, urgent referral to a regional cardiac unit is necessary for further investigation and probable surgical repair.

Atrio-ventricular (AV) canal

In the complete form of this condition, often seen in infants with Down's syndrome a common AV valve straddles a VSD combined with an ASD. In the partial form (the so-called ostium primum ASD), there is an ASD usually combined with a mitral valve abnormality causing mitral incompetence (MI).

Patients with an AV canal often present in the early neonatal period with heart failure, but with an ostium primum defect all that may be detected is a systolic murmur radiating into the axilla — suggesting MI.

CXR: Shows a large heart and pulmonary plethora.

ECG: Characteristically shows extreme QRS left axis deviation with bi-ventricular hypertrophy.

Diagnosis

Confirmed echocardiographically.

Treatment

Control heart failure medically. Pulmonary artery banding may be necessary in early infancy to reduce pulmonary blood flow, but repair of the defect and AV valve reconstruction may also be attempted at this stage.

Truncus arteriosus

This defect consists of a single arterial trunk which leaves the heart usually through a tricuspid valve and supplies the aorta, one or two pulmonary arteries, and the coronary arteries. A VSD is always present. The infants are not usually cyanosed. The pulses are bounding because of the run-off to the lungs via the pulmonary artery. S_1 is normal with a loud single or split S_2. There is an ejection click in 95% of cases; a pansystolic murmur is heard at the left lower sternal edge, often followed by a soft (diagnostic) early diastolic murmur of truncal valve insufficiency.

CXR: Right aortic arch occurs in 25% of cases with moderate cardiomegaly; increased pulmonary vascularity usually without enlargement of the main pulmonary artery.

ECG: Normal axis, biventricular hypertrophy.

Diagnosis

The diagnosis is made by echocardiography.

Treatment

The present treatment for truncus arteriosus is total correction in early infancy, closing the VSD, detaching the pulmonary artery from the aorta and joining it by means of a conduit to the right ventricle.

Interrupted aortic arch/aortic atresia/critical aortic stenosis

The clinical features of these conditions are similar. They present with cardiac failure, a low-output state, hypotension and acidosis within the first 24 hours. All the pulses may be small in volume, but careful attention to which of the arm or superficial temporal pulses are present gives important clues to the diagnosis, and to the extent of the interruption in the aortic arch.

The liver is markedly enlarged; the second sound may be loud and single, and there may be nothing more than a non-specific ejection systolic murmur. In critical AS there is usually an aortic ejection click.

Diagnosis

This is made echocardiographically, by demonstrating the defects in the aortic valve or arch.

Treatment

Perfusion of the lower part of the body is dependent on a patent ductus. This should be maintained by an infusion of PGE_1 while the diagnosis is established. Surgical correction of an interrupted aortic arch carries a high mortality because of the associated VSD and subaortic stenosis, but in aortic stenosis a valvotomy should be performed.

Coarctation of aorta syndrome

This is a combination of coarctation, usually preductal, with a patent ductus and other defects such as a VSD, ASD or complete transposition of the great vessels.

The infant presents with cardiac failure usually after the first week. On examination, in addition to heart failure, a gallop rhythm with either no murmur, or the murmur of the coexistent lesion is heard; the femoral pulses may be absent or reduced, and vary from hour to hour, depending on the patency of the ductus arteriosus.

CXR: Large heart with pulmonary venous congestion.

ECG: Usually right ventricular hypertrophy only.

Treatment

Control the heart failure. If the infant's condition is poor, keep the ductus patent (to perfuse the lower half of his body) with i.v. PGE_1, and then investigate him with echocardiography and angiocardiography if necessary. Surgical correction of the coarctation is virtually always necessary in the neonatal period, but repair of the other defects can usually be deferred.

Hypoplastic left-heart syndrome

This presents with heart failure and a low output state (shock). The lesion consists of a small or absent mitral valve and ascending aorta with aortic stenosis or atresia and a tiny left-ventricular cavity. It is always fatal. At birth no abnormality is noted, but gross cardiac failure, poor pulses, shock and varying degrees of cyanosis appear by 24–48 hours of age, with death occuring at a mean of 5 days. A soft pulmonary flow murmur may be present and S_2 is single. There is usually an obvious gallop rhythm.

CXR: A large globular heart and pulmonary congestion.

ECG: Right axis deviation, right atrial hypertrophy, right ventricular hypertrophy with a qR pattern over the right precordial leads.

Heart failure in the neonate not due to congenital heart disease

The causes of this are outlined in Table 17.2, the most important being perinatal ischaemia leading to myocardial damage (p.124). This presents in the first few hours of life. Heart failure due to metabolic problems and AV malformations is more common in the first 2–3 days whereas that due to infection or primary myocardial disease can present at any stage in the neonatal period.

It is always important to exclude AV malformations, particularly in the liver and brain, as the cause of heart failure. In such cases there is usually a loud systolic bruit over the organ in question, and malformations in the CNS can be demonstrated with ultrasound.

Treatment of heart failure in the neonate

1 Correct all associated biochemical abnormalities. If necessary give oxygen and bicarbonate, or ventilate the baby to control the blood gases.
2 Restrict the fluid intake to 100–120 ml/kg/24 hours; give less if the heart failure is severe.

Table 17.2. Causes of heart failure *not* due to congenital heart disease.

Severe birth asphyxia
Hypoglycaemia
Hypocalcaemia
Metabolic acidaemia
AV malformations
Glycogen storage disease
Myocarditis — Coxsackie
Thyrotoxicosis
Hydrops and all its causes (p.319)
Electrolyte disturbance, ↑ K, ↓ K, ↓ Na
Septicaemia
Anaemia
Primary cardiomyopathy, e.g. endocardial fibroelastosis

3 If the infant is very ill, maintain hydration intravenously, if he is not seriously ill but is unable to suck, he can be tube-fed.

4 Maintain blood pressure and volume by transfusion of plasma or blood: transfuse carefully under central venous pressure control, if possible, in infants suspected of having myocardial damage.

5 If heart failure is due to defective myocardial function, give dopamine or adrenalin by infusion.

6 Diuretics: frusemide 1 mg/kg b.d.; stat doses of up to 5 mg may be required initally. Check the electrolytes particularly in preterm infants on maintenance treatment.

7 Digoxin; the use of this drug is controversial. However, it should be used if heart failure does not respond to the therapy outlined above. Digitalize, giving the smaller dose intravenously with $5-7$ μg/kg $4-6$ times/24 hours. Maintain with 10 μg/kg/24 hours orally; measure plasma levels.

Cyanotic congenital heart disease

Differential diagnosis from pulmonary disease

History

1 Is the infant preterm and at risk from RDS?
2 Has he inhaled meconium?
3 Is there anything predisposing him to infection and pneumonia?

Examination

1 Dyspnoea. In pulmonary disease retraction, recession or grunting are usually present; with cyanotic CHD although there may be some tachypnoea from heart failure, dyspnoea is minimal.
2 Apnoea, hypotension, hypotonia are much more likely in sepsis or those forms of CHD associated with shock.
3 Cyanosis. In RDS the infant has a plethoric purplish cyanosis; in CHD the cyanosis is often 'slaty grey'.
4 Murmurs or heart failure (see above) strongly suggest CHD except where a PDA coexists with RDS (p.139).

Investigation

1 Check the blood gases: a P_aCO_2 >8 kPa (60 mmHg) strongly suggests lung disease. Give the infant 100% oxygen to breathe for 15 minutes to wash nitrogen out of his alveoli (hyperoxia test). In cyanotic CHD the P_aO_2 usually stays less than 6−7 kPa (45−50 mmHg) and always less than 13.3 kPa (100 mmHg).
2 Is there a low white count, or are bacteria demonstrated on a Gram stain of gastric aspirate suggesting sepsis (p.175)?
3 Is an L:S ratio (pp.33−4) on the mothers liquor or tracheal aspirate negative, suggesting RDS?
4 CXR:
  a Lung disease — parenchymal changes, normal heart size.
  b Sepsis — may be normal, pneumonia, or mild non-specific changes.
  c CHD — cardiomegaly; increase or decrease in vascularity
5 Is the ECG abnormal? Infants with respiratory disease usually have normal ECGs.
If cyanotic CHD is a possibility, further assessment by echocardiography proceeding, if necessary, to cardiac catheterization is mandatory.

Persistent fetal circulation (persistent transitional circulation, persistent pulmonary hypertension of the newborn)

This condition, which is not really true congenital heart disease, is due to pulmonary hypertension persisting after delivery, with the foramen ovale and the ductus arteriosus staying patent. The circulation of the blood through the heart and great vessels is therefore virtually identical to the fetal pattern. The condition is seen primarily in term infants. In some, no trigger is found, but in others the condition is provoked by perinatal hypoxia. Identical cardiovascular changes may develop secondary to severe neonatal lung disease such as RDS, meconium aspiration or GBS septicaemia.

Persistent fetal circulation (PFC) presents in the first few hours of life with marked cyanosis, but with minimal signs of respiratory distress, unless it is secondary to severe lung disease. The pulses and heart sounds are variable, though the pulmonary second sound may be loud; 50% of cases have a soft systolic murmur of tricuspid incompetence; cardiac failure is rare. Apart from profound hypoxaemia (P_aO_2 6–7 kPa [45–50 mmHg] in 100% oxygen) the blood gases are normal.

CXR: Often normal, but some patchy shadows may be seen, and the cardiothoracic ratio may be slightly increased.

ECG: Usually within normal limits.

Diagnosis

Echocardiographic demonstration of a normal heart excludes CHD and thereby establishes this diagnosis.

Treatment

Correct coexisting biochemical abnormalities, then try to set in train the normal postnatal changes in the circulation (p.38) by first lowering the pulmonary artery pressure. To do this ventilate the infant in 95% oxygen if necessary, and give a bolus of 1–2 mg of tolazoline intravenously, followed by an infusion of 2 mg/kg/hour. Alternatively, hyperventilate the infant to keep his P_aCO_2 in the range 3.3–4.0 kPa (25–30 mmHg) and his pH >7.5, since this also dilates the pulmonary arteries.

Cyanotic CHD due to structural defects (Table 17.3)

PULMONARY ATRESIA WITH INTACT VENTRICULAR SEPTUM

These babies usually have some degree of hypoplasia of the right ventricle and tricuspid valve. They present with cyanosis from birth which deepens over the first week depending on the flow through the ductus. The respiratory rate is increased, there is a prominent 'A' wave in the jugular veins, and over half the infants develop heart

Table 17.3. Cyanotic CHD due to structural defects. (From Cooke & Wilkinson, 1986, with permission.)

	Tachypnoea/dyspnoea	Pulses	Murmur	ECG	CXR
Transposition	Mild	Normal	None or ejection systolic 2–3/6	Upright T_3 in V_{3R} and V_1 (may be normal)	Heart normal or large (egg); mild to moderate plethora
Pulmonary atresia	Mild	Normal	Systolic 1–3/6 sometimes continuous 1–2/6	Axis $0°$ to $+60°$; RA+ Reduced RV	Large heart (RA+ LV+); oligaemic lungs
Fallot	Mild	Normal	Systolic 1–3/6 (ejection)	Often normal in newborn period	Normal or small heart; uptilted apex; oligaemic lungs; right aortic arch in 20%
Tricuspid atresia	Mild	Normal	Systolic 1–3/6 (ejection)	RA+; left axis deviation ($0°$ to $-90°$) LV+ Reduced RV.	Normal-sized heart; rather square; oligaemic lungs
TAPVD (obstructed)	Severe	Normal or small	None	RV+	Normal or small heart; lungs congested +++

failure. Auscultation reveals a single second sound; a systolic murmur is often heard due to a PDA or, since the only way out of the right ventricle is back through the tricuspid valve, to tricuspid incompetence.

ECG: Normal or rightward axis and right atrial hypertrophy, with primarily left ventricular forces on the chest leads.

CXR: Heart size depends on the degree of right atrial dilatation secondary to tricuspid incompetence, but is usually normal. The pulmonary artery shadow is absent, and the lung fields oligaemic.

Diagnosis

Echocardiography usually demonstrates an imperforate pulmonary valve, and almost always shows a thick-walled right ventricle with a small cavity and a small tricuspid valve.

Treatment

In the neonate, palliation by pulmonary valvotomy and some form of aorticopulmonary anastomosis such as a Blalock-Taussig shunt should be carried out. While the child is being prepared for this procedure an infusion of PGE_1 should be given to keep the ductus open, since this is the only route by which blood may reach the lungs. Subsequent correction depends on how well the right ventricle develops.

TRICUSPID ATRESIA

There is no tricuspid valve, and the floor of the right atrium is always muscular. Since the great vessels originate from appropriate ventricles, the pulmonary artery is supplied by left ventricular blood passing through a usually restrictive VSD into the rudimentary right ventricle and out through the pulmonary valve.

The S_2 is single, there are giant jugular 'A' waves, and usually an enlarged liver. There is almost always an ejection systolic murmur at the left sternal edge.

CXR: A square heart with cardiac enlargement in proportion to pulmonary blood flow; the pulmonary artery is absent and the lung fields are oligaemic.

ECG: Right atrial hypertrophy with left axis deviation and left ventricular hypertrophy manifest by a dominant S wave in the right precordial leads.

Diagnosis

Echocardiography demonstrates absence of the tricuspid valve and a small right ventricle.

Treatment

An aortico-pulmonary shunt (Blalock−Taussig) should be done early, proceeding to a right atrial−pulmonary artery conduit later in childhood.

TOTAL ANOMALOUS PULMONARY VENOUS DRAINAGE (OBSTRUCTED TYPE)

This is usually due to the pulmonary veins draining into the hepatic portal vein. This causes early cyanosis, heart failure and feeding difficulties. Babies with the non-obstructed type, usually draining somewhere above the diaphragm, do not become cyanosed, and present as heart failure during the second and third month. Obstructed babies have a loud first heart sound, fixed splitting of the second sound and often third and fourth heart sounds. Murmurs are rarely heard.

CXR: A small heart with severe pulmonary venous congestion.

ECG: Marked right ventricular and right atrial hypertrophy with right axis deviation.

Diagnosis

Echocardiography shows an increased right ventricular volume, a small left atrium and ventricle, and an echo-free space behind the left atrial wall. The anomalous common pulmonary vein and its course can be demonstrated.

Treatment

Surgical treatment should be carried out once the diagnosis is made.

TRANSPOSITION OF THE GREAT VESSELS

The aorta arises from the right ventricle, and the pulmonary artery from the left ventricle. This results in cyanosis, the intensity of which is dependent on whether or not there are associated shunts through a patent ductus or septal defects. In the absence of a VSD, the S_2 is often single but murmurs are often absent. Heart failure is common.

ECG: Right axis deviation and moderate right ventricular hypertrophy.

CXR: Egg-shaped heart with a narrow base and pulmonary plethora in 25% of cases, otherwise non-specific cardiac enlargement.

Diagnosis

The echocardiogram, demonstrating the origin of the high arching aorta from the right ventricle and bifurcating pulmonary artery from the left ventricle, is diagnostic.

Treatment

These infants survive due to the presence of circulatory mixing through the patent ductus or a septal defect. As soon as the diagnosis is made, the infant should receive intravenous prostaglandin E_1 to sustain ductal patency, until a palliative balloon atrial septostomy can be carried out to increase mixing between the systemic and pulmonary circulation.

Later in life the condition can be 'corrected' either by constructing an intra-atrial baffle to divert pulmonary venous blood through the tricuspid valve into the right ventricle and thence into the aorta and the systemic circulation, or more recently, by switching the arteries to their correct position.

TETRALOGY OF FALLOT

This condition is a combination of a large sub-aortic VSD, pulmonary and right ventricular infundibular stenosis and right ventricular hypertrophy. The degree of cyanosis depends on the severity of the right ventricular outflow tract stenosis, and thus on the size of the right-to-left shunt through the VSD. Cyanosis may be present from birth and deepen on crying. There is a systolic ejection murmur which tends to diminish with progressive infundibular narrowing during infancy, and may disappear completely during 'cyanotic spells', when the RV outflow tract contracts down.

The S_2 may be split with mild pulmonary valve obstruction, but is usually single.

CXR: Normal cardiothoracic ratio, decreased pulmonary vascularity without enlargement of the main pulmonary artery.

ECG: Right axis deviation, right ventricular hypertrophy with an upright T wave in V_1.

Diagnosis

This can usually be made on the basis of the clinical features, the chest X-ray, the ECG and the echocardiogram.

Treatment

In severe cases the ductus arteriosus should be kept patent with PGE_1 until a Blalock–Taussig shunt can be performed. Total correction can be carried out later in infancy.

Neonatal arrhythmias

These may be recognized *in utero*, and transplacental pharmacological control of tachycardias has been successful.

Atrial ectopics

These are common and do not require treatment.

Paroxysmal supraventricular tachycardia

This is the most common rhythm disorder in neonates. During attacks the heart rate may exceed 300/minute, with a normal QRS complex but no P waves; some will have Wolff–Parkinson–White syndrome on ECG; the episodes usually begin and end abruptly.

The child presents with irritability, poor feeding and the signs of heart failure. The diagnosis is made from the ECG. Death from heart failure may occur within 48–72 hours. 20% of babies will have repeated attacks.

Treatment

Stimulation of the vagus nerve by ducking the baby's face into ice-cold water for 5-10 seconds should be attempted. If this does not work, he should be digitalized and the above manoeuvres repeated. Once started, digoxin should be maintained for 6-12 months. In resistant cases, DC shock or i.v. verapamil may be needed.

Nodal and ventricular arrhythmias

Occasional nodal or ventricular ectopics are normal in neonates. Multiple ventricular ectopics, ventricular tachycardia and ventricular fibrillation signify serious cardiac or metabolic disease (acidaemia, hyperkalaemia, endotoxaemia) which require urgent treatment, and are often fatal.

Congenital heart block

30% of cases of complete or third degree congenital heart block have CHD, and those with a structurally normal heart are often delivered to mothers suffering from systemic lupus.

The infants present with bradycardia, often noted *in utero*, or cardiac failure. There may be an ejection murmur or a diastolic murmur even in the absence of structural defects.

Many infants are asymptomatic, and do not require treatment. Symptomatic cases, usually those with heart rates less than 50/minute and heart failure, require treatment with Isoprenaline to raise the heart rate to about 80/minute, followed by insertion of a pacemaker.

Further reading

Rowe, R.D., Freedom, R.M., Mehrizi, A. & Bloom, K.R. (1981) *The Neonate With Congenital Heart Disease*. W.B. Saunders Co., Philadelphia.
Wilkinson, J.L. & Cooke, R.W.I. (1986) Cardiovascular disorders. In *Textbook of Neonatology*, N.R.C. Roberton (ed.), Churchill Livingstone, Edinburgh. pp.340-82.

17.14

Chapter 18
Neurological Disease in the Newborn

Neonatal convulsions

The incidence of neonatal fits is hard to determine because subtle seizures may pass unnoticed, but is probably about 5:1000. It is important to recognize them, establish their cause and treat them promptly because:

1 Convulsions are usually related to significant illness.
2 Continuing seizure activity may, *per se*, lead to brain injury.

Types of convulsions

Neonatal convulsions differ from those seen in older children and adults. The classic tonic-clonic fit is seldom seen. Neonatal seizures are usually:

1 *Tonic*: with extension of limbs accompanied by other manifestations, e.g. deviation or jerking of the eyes, stertorous breathing or apnoea.
2 *Multifocal*: which progress in a random fashion quite unlike the orderly Jacksonian progression.
3 *Focal clonic*: well-localized clonic jerking.
4 *Subtle seizures*: these are likely to be missed and consist of one or more of the following:
 a Deviation or jerking of the eyes.
 b Repetitive blinking or sucking.
 c Tonic posturing of a limb.
 d Rhythmic 'swimming' movements of the arms or 'pedalling' of the legs.
5 *Apnoea*: usually with, but occasionally without, the above manifestations.

Jitteriness

This phenomenon, consisting of rapid tremulous movements of the limbs, can be mistaken for fits; Table 18.1 lists the distinguishing features.

208

Table 18.1.   Some distinguishing features of jitteriness versus seizures.

	Jitteriness	Seizures

Type of movement	Tremulous, fast
	Approximately 10/second
	Low amplitude
	Active contraction in both
	   phases of the movement
		Clonic jerking
		Slow 2–3/second
		Usually sluggish amplitude
		Contraction of agonists
		   with passive relaxation

Gaze	Normal	Frequently abnormal eye movements
Response to passive flexion	Usually cease	No response
Sensitivity to stimulus	Easily provoked	Usually not provoked

Aetiology (Table 18.2)

The most important and common causes are:
1 Hypoxic ischaemic encephalopathy with or without haemorrhage (see p.219).
2 Subarachnoid (p.214) or periventricular haemorrhage (p.215).
3 Metabolic disturbances (hypoglycaemia (p.269), hypocalcaemia (p.236), hypo- and hypernatraemia).
4 Bacterial meningitis (p.179).

Diagnosis

The cause of the fits can usually be established quite easily by taking a history of the perinatal period and the baby's subsequent progress, examining the infant and doing the following investigations:
1 Blood gases.
2 Blood glucose, electrolytes, calcium, magnesium, bilirubin.
3 Hb, WBC and differential.
4 Blood culture.
5 Lumbar puncture.
6 Cranial ultrasound scan.
These will establish a diagnosis in most cases. If the tests are negative and the fits are severe or there is persisting neurological abnormality, consider EEG, CT scan or investigation for the rare inborn errors of metabolism (Chapter 23).

Table 18.2 Differential diagnosis of neonatal convulsions.

Cause	Gestational age	Age (days)	Type of fit	Other features
Birth asphyxia (hypoxia, ischaemia trauma)	All	0–3	Any type	Antepartum and intrapartum history, fetal distress
Postnatal hypoxia	All	Any	Any type	Sick infant, following hypoxic episode
Intracranial haemorrhage				
Subdural	Mature	0–3	Any type	Traumatic delivery; now rare
Subarachnoid	Mature	0–3	Any type	Uniformly blood-stained CSF
Periventricular	<30 weeks	0–3	Usually tonic	History of birth or postnatal asphyxia; ultrasound confirms
Metabolic disturbance				
Hypoglycaemia	All	0–2	Clonic Apnoea	SFD, premature, maternal diabetes
Early hypocalcaemia	Prem.	0–2	Clonic/tonic	Usually sick infant
Late hypocalcaemia	Mature	>5	Multifocal	Usually well baby, high phosphate intake
Hypomagnesaemia	Mature	>5	Multifocal	Usually with hypocalcaemia
Hypernatraemia	Prem.	Any	Clonic	Dehydration, excess sodium intake
Hyponatraemia	Prem.	Any	Clonic	Oedema, fluid overload, inadequate Na intake
Hyperbilirubinaemia	Prem.	0–5	Any	Severe jaundice, ill, acidaemia
Inborn metabolic error (very rare)	Mature	0–3	Any	Lack of perinatal complications, +ve FH
Infective				
Meningitis	All	Any	Any	Other signs of sepsis
Congenital	All	Any	Any	SFD, multisystem disease
Drug withdrawal	All	0–5	Clonic	Maternal history
Idiopathic	All	Any	Any	Exclude other causes

Management

1 Sustain the airway if the infant is apnoeic/cyanotic or bradycardic. Start IPPV if necessary.
2 Do a Dextrostix, if <1.4 mmol/l do a formal blood glucose. Set up an intravenous infusion and give 0.5−1 g/kg dextrose (5−10 ml 10%) as a bolus and continue at 0.5 g/kg/hour.
3 Control the fits with the following (in order of preference):
  a Diazepam 1−2 mg/kg i.v. (NB this is often not effective).
  b Phenobarbitone 10−20 mg/kg i.v., repeated once if necessary.
  c Paraldehyde 0.5 ml/kg rectally or i.m. (NB very irritant drug).
  d Phenytoin 10 mg/kg i.v. repeated once if necessary.
  e Clormethiazole as infusion (0.6 ml/kg/hour of 8% solution, increasing as necessary).
4 Carry out the investigations listed above.
5 Treat the underlying illness — if possible:
  a Hypoxic ischaemic encephalopathy with cerebral oedema (p.125).
  b Meningitis (p.179).
  c Electrolyte or metabolic error (Chapter 23).
  d PVH — no treatment possible (p.217).

Maintenance therapy

This is always necessary unless the fits were brief and due to some transient and treatable cause, e.g. hypoglycaemia, hypocalcaemia. Phenobarbitone is the drug of choice (5 mg/kg/day). If the fits are easily-controlled and the infant becomes neurologically normal over the ensuing week or two it is reasonable to reduce the dose and then stop altogether. When fits have been very severe or the infant remains neurologically abnormal, more prolonged therapy is indicated.

Prognosis

The following are guidelines:

Good prognosis. Fits due to mild birth asphyxia, subarachnoid haemorrhage, hypocalcaemia.

Guarded prognosis. Severe birth asphyxia (p.125), intraventricular or intracerebral haemorrhage (p.219), prolonged hypoglycaemia, hypo- or hyper-natraemia, meningitis.

Poor prognosis. Any condition in which the infant remains neurologically abnormal for a prolonged period; cerebral malformation.

The floppy infant

The common causes are prematurity and/or CNS depression; rarer causes include spinal cord injury, hereditary neuropathy or myopathy and metabolic disorders. Hypotonia is also characteristic of certain syndromes, e.g. Down's, Prader—Willi. Hypotonic infants look very much the same irrespective of aetiology, lying in a frog-like posture with little or no resistance to passive movements.

Evaluation

1 Ask about fetal movements during pregnancy.
2 Assess muscle strength by:
  a Observing anti-gravity movements.
  b Pulling the infant up by his wrists and observing the degree of head lag.
  c Observing whether the limbs hang limply with the infant held in ventral suspension.
3 Observe facial movement, mobility and the strength of the cry.
4 Palpate the skeletal muscles for bulk and do the reflexes.
This examination usually places the baby into one of two broad groups:

Non-paralytic

Hypotonia but little or no weakness. These babies can move their limbs against gravity either spontaneously or in response to a stimulus.

Paralytic

Weakness and hypotonia in proportion; anti-gravity movements are poor or absent. These infants may be severely hypotonic with cranial nerve involvement as well as skeletal muscle weakness. They may have difficulty in sucking and swallowing and become apnoeic.

Aetiology and differential diagnosis (non-paralytic)

The non-paralytic causes of hypotonia are by and large the causes of severe illness in the neonatal period:
• Prematurity

- Drug depression
- Birth asphyxia
- RDS
- Septicaemia
- Intracranial haemorrhage
- Metabolic disturbance
- Dysmorphic syndromes
- Congenital hypothyroidism (rare)
- Connective tissue disorders, (e.g. Ehlers–Danlos syndrome)

Aetiology and differential diagnosis (paralytic)

This includes the serious acquired and inherited disorders of nerve and muscle.

Spinal cord injury (p.223).

Anterior horn cell disease

Congenital spinal muscular atrophy (Werdnig–Hoffman disease). Inherited as a recessive. Profound hypotonia and weakness; tendon reflexes are absent; fasciculation of the tongue may be seen. Diagnosis confirmed by muscle biopsy, prognosis bad.

Congenital poliomyelitis. This is very rare.

Neuromuscular junction disorders

Neonatal myasthenia gravis is rare and presents within 3 days of birth; the mother is usually affected. Cranial nerve disturbances common with facial weakness. Diagnosis confirmed by improvement following injection of edrophonium 0.2 mg/kg i.m. (tensilon test).

Muscle disorders

Dystrophia myotonica. Affected neonates are markedly hypotonic. Autosomal dominant; but only babies of affected mothers present neonatally. Diagnosis is by examining the mother for myotonia and enquiring about a family history of early onset cataracts and premature balding.

Congenital myopathies. Several rare, mostly autosomal recessive primary muscle disorders may present in the neonatal period. Muscle biopsy and sophisticated histochemistry are essential to sort them out.

Congenital muscular dystrophy. This heterogeneous group has a similar clinical picture to the primary myopathies but the aetiology is less clear-cut.

Metabolic disorders. The best known example is glycogen storage disease type II (Pompe's disease) inherited as an autosomal recessive.

Other causes of hypotonia

It is not always possible to ascertain the cause of neonatal hypotonia, and there remains a group assigned to the rather unsatisfactory diagnosis 'benign congenital hypotonia'.

Intracranial haemorrhage and hypoxic ischaemic encephalopathy

Haemorrhagic and ischaemic lesions of the CNS are now the most important causes of neonatal death and are responsible for the majority of handicap among survivors. Factors influencing cerebral blood flow (CBF, Fig. 18.1), are of key importance in understanding the aetiology of these lesions.

CBF is largely independent of systemic blood pressure under physiological conditions. Asphyxia leads to loss of so-called 'autoregulation' so that CBF becomes pressure passive. Hypercapnia and hypoxia are cerebral vasodilators, whereas hypocapnia and hyperoxia result in vasoconstriction.

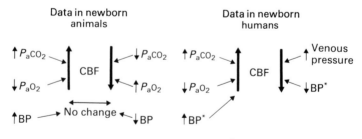

Fig. 18.1. Factors known to influence cerebral blood flow in the neonate. (From Pape & Wigglesworth, 1979.)

Subdural haemorrhage

See birth trauma, p.222.

Subarachnoid haemorrhage

This is the commonest haemorrhage in mature infants and is of venous origin; it is primarily due to asphyxia with or without minor trauma and does not present the dramatic picture seen in adults. Babies with subarachnoid haemorrhage may:
1 Be completely asymptomatic.
2 Be irritable, presumably with a headache.
3 Have fits (p.210).
Unless associated with severe asphyxia, such infants are usually remarkably well. Diagnosis is by finding uniformly bloody CSF. The prognosis for normal development is excellent; very rarely, hydrocephalus develops due to obliterative arachnoiditis.

Periventricular/intraventricular haemorrhage (PVH)

PVH is the commonest form of intracranial haemorrhage in the newborn. Ultrasound and CT scans show an incidence which is inversely related to weight and GA (Table 18.3). However, only a minority are clinically significant. The preferred nomenclature for all lesions is PVH, although if the haemorrhage is clearly limited within the ventricle, it may be described as an IVH.

Table 18.3. Incidence of periventricular haemorrhage (PVH) of all types.

By birthweight (kg)				
Birthweight	<1.0	1.0−1.5	1.5−2.0	>2.0
% with PVH	43	19	6	0.01

By gestational age (weeks)					
Gestational age	<26	27−28	29−30	31−32	>32
% with PVH	86	50	36	30	7

Pathophysiology

The basic lesion is haemorrhage into the prominent subependymal germinal matrix overlying the caudate nucleus in the premature infant. There are three crucial factors in the development of PVH:
1 The fragile and poorly-supported immature capillaries of the ger-

minal layer are especially prone to rupture during surges of blood flow.

2 A major proportion of CBF is directed to the basal ganglia and germinal layer. Thus factors which increase it such as decreased P_aO_2 or increased P_aCO_2 may predispose towards PVH.

3 Cerebral blood flow may become *pressure passive* due to loss of autoregulation. Systemic hypotension may then cause brain ischaemia, and hypertension may cause haemorrhage in the fragile germinal layer.

Thus, intrapartum asphyxia (especially breech extraction), or acute postnatal asphyxia (e.g. an apnoeic attack, a blocked endotracheal tube or a pneumothorax in babies on IPPV for RDS), which can cause either sudden increases in CBF by lowering P_aO_2 and/or raising P_aCO_2 and BP, or hypotension and thus cerebral ischaemia, predispose to PVH.

Classification

Germinal layer haemorrhage (GLH) or subependymal haemorrhage (SEH). Haemorrhage confined to the subependymal germinal layer, i.e no blood within the ventricles = grade 1.

Intraventricular haemorrhage (IVH). Haemorrhage which ruptures through the ependyma into the lateral ventricles. This may only be a small leak with no ventricular distension (grade 2), or it may extend to fill and distend the whole ventricular system (grade 3).

Intracerebral haemorrhage, extends beyond the ventricles into the white matter (grade 4). This is true periventricular haemorrhage.

It is not always easy to separate grades 1, 2, and 3 on the basis of ultrasound.

Clinical picture

Asymptomatic. Small GLHs are asymptomatic and are only diagnosed by routine ultrasound. Even quite large PVHs may occur without clinical signs.

Catastrophic. A sudden and dramatic deterioration with cardio-respiratory collapse (apnoea, bradycardia, pallor, hypotension, peripheral vascular shutdown). Hypotonia, tonic seizures and general unresponsiveness develop. Blood gases show hypoxia and acidaemia; the PCV falls.

More subtle deterioration. A more gradual decline in the infant's general condition (over hours or days) with apnoeic/bradycardic episodes, fits, reduced motor activity and responsiveness, acidaemia, anaemia and the need for increased ventilatory support.

Diagnosis

This is made by cranial ultrasound. Clinical deterioration due to PVH has to be differentiated from:
- Worsening RDS, pneumothorax, etc.
- Infection
- Other causes of anaemia (p.286)
- Other causes of convulsions (p.210)

Evolution of PVH

Fifty per cent of PVHs occur on day 1. Haemorrhage arising *de novo* is rare after 4 days. Small GLHs without other complications usually resolve spontaneously, Massive intraventricular or intracerebral bleeds associated with clinical deterioration are often rapidly fatal. With moderate haemorrhage or following successful resuscitation the blood is gradually resorbed over the next few days or weeks.

Prevention

Try to avoid risk factors by:
1 Careful antenatal monitoring to detect fetal distress.
2 Delivery by caesarean section with:
 a breech presentation <32 weeks.
 b significant antepartum haemorrhage.
3 Swift, efficient resuscitation at birth.
4 Avoiding postnatal asphyxial episodes.
5 Avoiding rapid and large postnatal swings in blood pressure.

Management once PVH occurs

1 Maintain cerebral perfusion by correcting hypotension with plasma or blood (if the PCV is low); After volume correction use a dopamine infusion if hypotension persists.

2 Avoid hypercapnia and hypoxia.
3 Maintain glucose and electrolyte homeostasis.
4 Monitor the haemorrhage by serial ultrasound, and measure the head circumference daily.

Progressive ventricular dilatation

This may be due to cerebral atrophy or to obstructed CSF circulation following the haemorrhage. Dilatation precedes increase in head size by days or weeks. To deal with this problem consider:

Serial lumbar punctures. If CSF pathways are not blocked in the posterior fossa it may be possible to remove ventricular CSF at lumbar puncture.

Ventriculostomy with open drainage. This may be a useful temporary measure if the CSF protein is >10 g/l, but there is a danger of infection.

Insertion of an indwelling reservoir. This can be tapped as required through the skin, but may be difficult to insert in tiny infants.

Drugs to reduce CSF production. Acetazolamide, glycerol and isosorbide have been used with limited success.

Shunting procedures. Ventriculo-atrial or ventriculo-peritoneal shunts may be needed if the above measures fail to prevent progressive hydrocephalus.

Prognosis

The prognosis for infants with GLHs is the same as that with no haemorrhage. For infants with large intracerebral bleeds the initial mortality is high (50–75%) and virtually all the survivors are handicapped. The morbidity is probably more related to ischaemia and the later development of periventricular leucomalacia (PVL, p.219). For infants with intraventricular or small intracerebral lesions the outlook is reasonable, very few survivors being severely handicapped. Hydrocephalus, if adequately treated, does not itself significantly alter the outcome.

Hypoxic ischaemic encephalopathy (HIE)

This is a major cause of both mortality and morbidity. The primary factor is *hypoxia* of brain tissue which arises either from hypoxaemia or ischaemia due to inadequate perfusion; these two factors usually coexist.

Arterial blood supply to the brain

There are two basic systems:
1 An 'external' system with arterial branching from the surface towards the centre (ventriculopetal).
2 An 'internal' system branching from the centre of the cerebrum towards the periphery (ventriculofugal).
These produce 'watershed' zones between the different arterial territories, and are the areas most susceptible to *ischaemic* damage.

Causes of HIE

- Perinatal asphyxia
- Severe respiratory disease
- Severe apnoeic attacks
- Severe cardiac failure
- Vascular collapse associated with haemorrhage, fluid loss or sepsis

Neuropathology and clinical correlations

Various patterns of brain injury are described neuropathologically (Table 18.4). The term infant with severe CNS involvement following birth asphyxia (p.124) usually suffers selective neuronal necrosis, whereas the asphyxiated preterm infant develops PVL. Recent work suggests that haemorrhage into PVL is an important component in the development of grade 4 intracerebral PVH (see above).

See Chapter 14 for clinical picture and management of HIE in the term infant. The prevention and treatment of HIE in the preterm infant is that outlined above for PVH.

Birth injury

This is now rare due to improved obstetric care.

Table 18.4 Topography, neonatal picture and long-term sequelae of various types of hypoxic ischaemic injury.

Lesion	Topography	Neonatal picture	Long-term sequelae
Selective neuronal necrosis (hypoxic)	Cerebral and cerebellar cortex, thalamus, brainstem motor nuclei	Stupor/coma, seizures, hypotonia, sucking/swallowing disturbance	Mental retardation, spastic quadriplegia, convulsions, ataxia ? hyperactivity
Status marmoratus (hypoxic)	Basal ganglia, thalamus	Unknown (rare)	Choreoathetosis, spastic quadriplegia
Parasaggital cerebral injury	Cerebral cortex posterior> anterior, watershed infarcts	Asphyxiated mature infants, proximal limb weakness	Spastic quadriparesis/hemiparesis ? intellectual deficits
Periventricular leucomalacia (ischaemic)	Periventricular white matter	Premature: ? lower limb weakness	Spastic diplegia, intellectual deficits
Focal ischaemic necrosis	Cortex and subcortical white matter, porencephaly	Variable, hemiplegia, quadriplegia	Spastic, hemi/quadriparesis, convulsions

Predisposing factors

- Cephalo-pelvic disproportion
- Prematurity
- Prolonged labour
- Posterior position
- Breech or compound presentation
- Rotational forceps
- Versions or extractions

Skull

The fetal head is liable to damage during delivery either from forceps or from pressure against the pelvis during labour.

Cephalhaematoma (Fig. 18.2)

This common injury consists of a subperiosteal haemorrhage over one or more of the skull bones limited by the suture lines, and occurs in 2–3% of all deliveries, being more common in primiparae; 33% are associated with forceps. Clinically, there is a fluctuant swelling over the affected bone which resolves over the next few weeks. No treatment is needed.

Subaponeurotic haemorrhage (subgaleal haemorrhage) (Fig. 18.2)

In this rare injury bleeding occurs over the whole scalp in the subaponeurotic layer.

Linear skull fractures

These are only likely to come to light if the skull is X-rayed for some other reason and are of no significance in themselves. Usually parietal; may be associated with cephalhaematoma or, very rarely, an extradural haemorrhage.

Depressed skull fractures

Occasionally, compressive forces acting on the skull result in a localized depressed fracture rather like pressing on a ping-pong ball. No treatment is needed if the infant is clinically well.

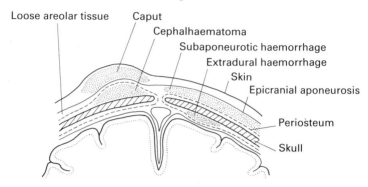

Fig. 18.2. Different types of scalp and skull injury. (From Pape & Wigglesworth, 1979.)

Subdural haemorrhage

This primarily traumatic lesion is now very rare and is almost confined to fullterm infants. It occurs when there is excessive moulding of the head during delivery, stretching the falx and tentorium and rupturing the dural sinuses; such injuries are most likely to occur with:
1 Gross cephalopelvic disproportion.
2 Malpresentation, e.g. breech, brow, face.
3 Difficult forceps delivery, e.g. Kielland's.
Small subdural haemorrhages do not need to be drained and large ones are usually associated with fatal hypoxic ischaemic encephalopathy. Specific treatment is therefore rarely indicated.

Facial nerve palsy

Injury to the facial nerve occurs as it emerges from the stylomastoid foramen and is caused by pressure from the maternal sacral promontory; it is seldom caused by forceps. Usually lower and upper face are involved but the palsy may not be obvious until the baby cries with a lop-sided mouth and fails to close one eye. Almost all recover spontaneously within a week or two.

Brachial plexus injury

Injury to the brachial plexus results from traction and lateral flexion of the neck. In vertex deliveries it arises during delivery of the shoulders and in breech deliveries during delivery of the head. There is often an associated fractured clavicle (p.296).

Clinical picture

The commonest form is Erb's palsy involving the upper plexus roots (C4, 5 and 6). The baby cannot abduct his shoulder, flex his elbow, supinate his forearm or extend his wrist (the 'waiters tip' position); a grasp reflex is, however, present. Much more rarely there is a total plexus palsy with paralysis of the intrinsic muscles of the hand in addition to the above abnormalities.

Treatment

None initially: if still present after 2 weeks, the baby should have physiotherapy to prevent joint contractures.

Prognosis

Outlook for spontaneous recovery is good (90% within a year and most within a few weeks).

Phrenic nerve palsy

The diaphragm is supplied predominantly from C4. Damage can be isolated to this root but is more often (90%) associated with Erb's palsy. Presents with tachypnoea, hypoxia and hypoventilation: diagnosed by fluoroscopy. Most recover spontaneously.

Treatment

That of the respiratory failure.

Spinal cord injury

This rare problem occurs following vaginal delivery of a breech with an extended neck. The infant has a flaccid quadriplegia which may affect the diaphragm. There is no treatment and the prognosis is poor.

Congenital abnormalities of the central nervous system

Neural tube defects (NTD)

Defects in neural tube closure occur anywhere along its length but are commonest in the fore brain (anencephaly) and in the thoraco-lumbar or lumbo-sacral region (myelomeningocele). The lesions vary between gross malformations to comparatively minor abnormalities entirely compatible with normal life.

Aetiology

This is multifactorial but poorly understood; NTDs are commonest among the Welsh and Irish, and the risk increases with decreasing social class. Hereditary factors also operate (p.227). There is considerable interest in the role of periconceptional nutritional deficiencies. The average UK incidence is now 1:1000 LB.

Anencephaly

The forebrain and calvarium are incompletely developed; the lesion is incompatible with life. Most cases are now diagnosed by early ultrasound and the pregnancy is terminated.

Cranium bifidum (encephalocele and meningocele)

Cerebral cortex and/or meninges protrude through a bony defect most commonly (75–80%) in the occipital region, and the lesions are usually skin-covered. Those containing only meninges and CSF (meningocele) have a good prognosis; more often they contain brain tissue and are associated with other intra-cranial dysgeneses and have a poor outlook.

Management

Ultrasound and/or CT scan are useful for assessment. Meningoceles and very small encephaloceles should be excised. Encephaloceles associated with neurological abnormalities should be treated symptomatically.

Spina bifida cystica

These lesions vary in size between comparatively small to those extending over many segments. A few, mainly meningoceles, are skin-covered. 94% are myelomeningoceles, only 6% being meningoceles. 80% involve the thoraco-lumbar, lumbar, or lumbo-sacral region.

Clinical features

Hydrocephalus due to the brain stem being jammed in the foramen magnum (Arnold–Chiari malformation) may be clinically evident at birth or may only become apparent later. There may be gross musculo-skeletal deformities secondary to partial paraplegia.

Thoraco-lumbar lesions usually result in total paraplegia without deformity; sacral lesions affect primarily the sphincters. Lumbo-sacral lesions vary depending on the segments involved. There are disturbances of bladder function in over 90% of cases. Lesions above the sacrum lead to automatic bladder emptying whereas those affecting primarily the sacral roots are associated with an atonic bladder and dribbling incontinence.

Assessment

The important points to note are:
1 Any other congenital abnormalities.
2 The size and site of the lesion.
3 The nature of the sac. Is it intact (or skin covered), or has it ruptured? Are neural elements visible?
4 Are there deformities such as kyphosis, scoliosis, dislocated hips, talipes?
5 Is there hydrocephalus? (OFC >90th centile). Measure the OFC and assess ventricular size with ultrasound.
6 Establish the sensory level to pinprick by, for example, noting facial expression; ignore a spinal withdrawal reflex.
7 Observe *spontaneous* movement of the legs. Ignore reflex movements in response to stimuli. A guide to the motor level is given in Fig. 18.3.

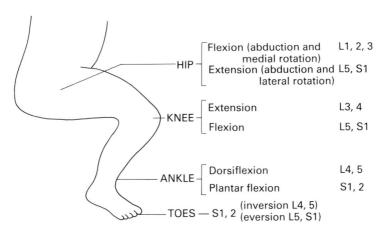

Fig. 18.3. The lower limb myotomes. (From Brocklehurst, 1976.)

8 Is the anal sphincter patulous? Is the bladder enlarged? Is there dribbling incontinence?

Complications

1 Infection. The exposed lesion is an open invitation to meningitis.
2 Hydrocephalus occurs in 80%.
3 Orthopaedic deformities secondary to neurological involvement.
4 Urological: incontinence, ureteric reflux, hydronephrosis, infection.
5 Bowel incontinence or constipation.
6 Mental retardation especially with hydrocephalus and ventriculitis.

Management

Assessment of long-term results of repairing the spinal defect immediately after delivery suggested that the following were contraindications to immediate surgery:
• Large defects
• High defects (L1 and above)
• High sensory level (above L1)
• Severe limb deformities
• Gross hydrocephalus at birth (head circumference >90th centile)
• Kyphosis or kyphoscoliosis
Infants with smallish defects and those in which limb movements are preserved should be operated on early to prevent entry of infection. For infants not operated on the lesion should be dressed and the baby fed and cared for normally; subsequent neurological, paediatric, urological and orthopaedic procedures are planned as the need arises.

Prognosis

More than half the cases will not be treated immediately and of these only about 10−20% will survive more than 1 year. The 5 year survival rate of infants selected for early closure is about 80% and of these two-thirds will be normal or have minimal impairment, one-third will have moderate disability (moderate motor defects and incontinence). Most survivors (in both groups) will require shunting for hydrocephalus in early infancy and complex orthopaedic and urological procedures in the subsequent months.

Talking to parents

This is covered in detail in Chapter 4. Clearly decisions about management must be taken only after prolonged discussion not only with the parents but also with their GP and other professionals.

Meningocele

When only meninges are involved the underlying spinal cord is intact. Most are skin-covered and require no immediate treatment. The sac can be excised later and the prognosis is excellent.

Genetic counselling

The chances of a recurrence following an affected pregnancy is about 4–5%. After 2 affected pregnancies the risk is 10–15%. All mothers with a family history of NTD should be offered antenatal detection.

Anencephaly and most neural tube defects can be detected by careful ultrasound examination of the fetus at 14–18 weeks. In addition the level of α-fetoprotein is raised in the liquor and in the plasma of mothers carrying an infant with an open NTD.

Other spinal dysraphisms

Any mid-line lesions overlying the spine should be regarded with suspicion. These include:
- Hairy patch
- Birthmark
- Lipoma
- Dermal sinus, particularly in the lumbo-sacral or occipital regions; small sacro-coccygeal pits are common and harmless

Any of these abnormalities may indicate not only vertebral anomalies, but also cord involvement. A dermal sinus may communicate with the dura with a consequent risk of meningitis. A lipoma may give rise to progressive disturbance due to tethering of the cord. Infants with suspicious lesions should be X-rayed, those with dermal sinuses or lipomata should be referred to the neurosurgeon.

Sacral agenesis (caudal regression syndrome)

This rare anomaly leading to atrophic changes in the bones and muscles of the legs and sphincter disturbances, has a strong association with maternal diabetes; 15% of cases occur in infants of diabetic mothers and the risk of a diabetic mother having an affected infant is approximately 0.5–1%.

Hydrocephalus

There are two types of hydrocephalus:

Obstructive (non-communicating)

Distension occurs proximal to a block in the ventricular system; the commonest site of obstruction is the aqueduct.

Communicating

The intraventricular pathways for CSF are open with dilatation of the entire ventricular system. The block lies in the subarachnoid space with either occlusion of the basal cisterns or obliteration of the subarachnoid space over the cerebral convexities.

Aetiology of obstructive hydrocephalus

1 Congenital aqueduct stenosis: the commonest cause of uncomplicated hydrocephalus, occasionally inherited as a sex-linked recessive.
2 Acquired stenosis following haemorrhage (p.218) or infection (p.180).
3 External compression of the aqueduct by cysts, vascular malformations, tumours, or haemorrhage into the posterior fossa.
4 Atresia of the foramina of Lushka and Magendie. This results in cystic dilatation of the fourth ventricle (Dandy–Walker malformation) and cerebellar malformation.

Aetiology of communicating hydrocephalus

1 Arnold–Chiari malformation (p.225).
2 Obliteration of the subarachnoid space following:
  a Haemorrhage (p.218).
  b Meningitis (p.180).
  c Congenital infections (p.184).
3 Encephalocele.
4 Congenital absence of arachnoid granulations.
5 Choroid plexus papilloma.

Diagnosis

May be obvious at birth with OFC >90th centile, large, tense anterior fontanelle, and splayed cranial sutures. Thereafter it becomes evident when the head enlarges abnormally rapidly. Diagnosis is by ultrasound.

Treatment

A cerebral mantle of <1 cm is a poor prognostic sign. Hydrocephalus without malformation has a 90% survival rate following CSF drainage by a ventriculo-peritoneal or right atrial shunt. Two-thirds of the survivors have an IQ >75.

Microcephaly

This is a head circumference more than 3 SD below the mean for GA. It may be primary or secondary.

Primary

1 Familial:
  a autosomal recessive.
  b sex-linked recessive.
2 Sporadic, idiopathic.
3 Teratogenic, e.g. radiation.

Secondary microcephaly

1 Intra-uterine infection with:
  a Cytomegalovirus.
  b Toxoplasma.
  c Rubella.
2 Chromosomal abnormalities.
3 Other CNS developmental disorders and syndromes.
4 Following severe perinatal insult (e.g. asphyxia, PVL, meningitis), in this case the microcephaly will only become obvious later.
Although microcephaly is untreatable, it is clearly important to establish a diagnosis because of the genetic and developmental implications.

Holoprosencephaly

This severe defect is often associated with mid-line facial anomalies (cleft palate, cyclopia, etc.). The cerebrum consists of a single sphere with a single mid-line cavity. The corpus callosum, basal ganglia and thalami are absent as are the olfactory bulbs and tracts (arrhinencephaly).

Diagnosis

By ultrasound or CT scan.

Hydranencephaly

The cerebral hemispheres are absent and replaced by a large fluid-filled cavity, although the brain stem and basal ganglia are well-formed. Aetiology is obscure. The infant may appear remarkably normal with appropriate reflex behaviour, but there is no visual following.

Diagnosis

By transillumination of the skull or by ultrasound.

References

Pape, K.E. & Wigglesworth, J.S. (1979) Haemorrhage, ischaemia and the perinatal brain. *Clinics in Developmental Medicine Nos. 69/70.* Heinemann Medical Books, London.
Brocklehurst, G. (1976) Spina bifida for the clinician. *Clinics in Developmental Medicine No. 57,* Heinemann Medical Books, London.

Further reading

Dubowitz, V. (1980) The floppy infant. *Clinics in Developmental Medicine No. 76.* Heinemann Medical Books, London.
Volpe, J.J. (1981) *Neurology of the Newborn.* W.B. Saunders Co., Philadephia.

Chapter 19
Fluid, Electrolyte and Acid Base Balance in the Sick Newborn

Water balance

Physiology

The glomerular filtration rate (GFR) averages $10-15$ ml/minute/1.73 m^2 in premature infants and $20-30$ ml/minute/1.73 m^2 in fullterm infants during the first few days, and reaches the adult $120-130$ ml/minute/1.73 m^2 by $6-12$ months. Urine production is $25-60$ ml/kg/24 hours in the neonatal period. The newborn infant, particularly if sick or born prematurely, has difficulty coping with either excess fluid or fluid deprivation. If more fluid than he needs is given, particularly intravenously, he cannot produce dilute urine, and will therefore become oedematous; conversely, if inadequately hydrated he cannot concentrate his urine beyond $600-700$ mOsmol/kg H_2O in the first month, so he becomes dehydrated more rapidly than a more mature infant.

Controlling water balance in sick neonates is difficult, and fluid overload or dehydration can develop easily and quickly. The serious consequences of both these problems are outlined below. However, these problems are limited to infants requiring intravenous fluids and are rare in those of all gestations who are well enough to be fed orally, although such infants can become dehydrated if insufficient fluid is given.

Fluid overload, fluid retention and oedema

These problems are easy to recognize if fluid retention is marked and oedema develops. However, the early stages of fluid retention are best detected by regularly weighing ill neonates. A normally hydrated baby, receiving only maintenance glucose electrolyte solution intravenously, should lose $1-2\%$ of his body weight daily. A static weight, or weight gain under these circumstances strongly suggests fluid retention.

Fluid overload may occur if:

1 Too much intravenous fluid is given for maintenance.

2 Boluses of bicarbonate, dextrose, plasma or blood are given without adjusting the maintenance fluid intake.

3 The rate rather than the concentration of solutions of glucose, bicarbonate or dopamine is increased if hypoglycaemia, acidaemia or hypotension persist.

4 Too much fluid is infused through umbilical catheters to clear them after samples have been taken.

5 The volume of fluid given as intravenous drugs (e.g. antibiotics, pancuronium) is not included in the daily intake.

6 There is mechanical failure or inaccurate setting of the drip controllers or infusion pumps.

Fluid retention occurs in infants with:

1 Asphyxia, hypotension, RDS, septicaemia, acidaemia, etc., who have damaged kidneys and/or leaky capillaries.

2 CNS damage (e.g. asphyxia, meningitis) causing inappropriate ADH secretion.

3 A rise in central venous pressure due to CPAP or IPPV + PEEP — probably mediated through increased ADH release.

4 Hypoalbuminaemia with fluid leaking in to the extracellular fluid.

Fluid overload and/or retention virtually always causes peripheral oedema, but in addition may cause:

1 Congestive heart failure, including left ventricular failure and massive pulmonary haemorrhage (p.157).

2 Pulmonary oedema exacerbating the hypoxaemia in all lung diseases.

3 An increased incidence of PDA in infants recovering from RDS (p.193).

4 An increased incidence of BPD (p.158).

5 Hyponatraemia, hypokalaemia.

6 Kidney, liver and gut oedema; making these organs less effective at excreting urine, conjugating drugs and bilirubin, and more prone to NEC.

7 Cerebral oedema — especially if there is coexistent brain damage from asphyxia or hypoxia.

8 Sclerema (p.182).

Clinical problems and their treatment

There are five common patterns of fluid retention and oedema encountered in sick neonates, most of whom are receiving their fluid intravenously. Each type of problem requires a different approach and management.

1 Fluid retention and oedema due to heart failure (p.193). Treat the condition causing the congestive cardiac failure: restrict intravenous fluids to 60−70 ml/kg/24 hours. Give diuretics and perhaps digoxin (p.199).

2 Oedema due to hypoalbuminaemia or hydrops. Treat any underlying illness; restrict the overall fluid intake to 50−60 ml/kg/24 hours. Infuse albumin, 0.5 g/kg, aiming to raise the plasma albumin above 20 g/l. Diuretics should be given after this infusion to prevent heart failure as fluid is drawn osmotically into the plasma.

3 Incorrect and inadvertent overadministration of fluid. Restrict the fluid to 30−40 ml/kg/24 hours and give frusemide 1.0 mg/kg i.v.

4 Oedema in seriously ill neonates who have leaky capillaries but do not have overt heart failure, hypoalbuminaemia or iatrogenic overhydration.

The typical infant suffering from this condition is preterm with RDS and is being treated with pancuronium while on IPPV and PEEP. Treatment is to restrict fluid to 60−70 ml/kg/24 hours with careful supervision of electrolytes, urinary output, blood pressure and peripheral perfusion. If oedema is a clinical problem, despite the absence of fluid overload a dose of Lasix, 1.0 mg/kg can be given intravenously.

5 Oedema due to inappropriate ADH secretion.

This is common in infants who have suffered neurological damage with meningitis or birth asphyxia. The infants have hyponatraemia, hypo-osmolality, and a low urinary output. A low serum osmolality with a urinary osmolality above 300 mOsmol/kgH$_2$O establishes the diagnosis. Treat by correcting the underlying problem plus strict fluid restriction to 30−40 ml/kg/24 hours.

Dehydration

This readily develops in neonates due to their inability to produce concentrated urine. It occurs in the following circumstances:

1 A high insensible water loss — over 100 ml/kg/24 hours with overhead radiant heaters.

2 An osmotic diuresis caused by glycosuria in infants <1.5 kg receiving high concentrations of Dextrose i.v.

3 Gut fluid loss in diarrhoea and vomiting.

4 Inadequate intake — i.v. tissued, fluid deliberately withheld to avoid overload!

5 Over-vigorous use of diuretics.

The effects of fluid loss are:

1 Reduction in the plasma volume leading to tissue hypoxia and acidaemia, gut under-perfusion predisposing to NEC, and compromised renal function with pre-renal uraemia, and ultimately severe dehydration and shock.

2 An increased incidence of jaundice (p.256).

3 Electrolyte abnormalities, particularly hypernatraemia which may cause neurological damage.

Dehydration in the neonate is easy to recognize with weight-loss, decreased skin turgor, sunken eyes and a depressed fontanelle.

Treatment

Give at least 150 ml of fluid/kg/24 hours; much larger volumes are often necessary to replace pre-existing fluid loss, or to keep up with continuing fluid loss in diarrhoea or vomiting.

With fever, increase i.v. fluid maintainance by 5−10 ml/kg/24 hours/°C above 37°C. To compensate for insensible water loss with overhead heaters, an extra 50−75 ml/kg/24 hours may be required.

Adding all these together the infant may need a total of 250−300 ml/kg/24 hours.

Maintenance fluid therapy

Sick neonates who need i.v. therapy for one reason or another should start on 60−80 ml/kg/24 hours. Initially, in both term and preterm infants, this should be given as 10% dextrose. Add electrolytes (Na, K, Cl, Ca) at some stage during the first 24−72 hours depending on the results of the daily electrolyte values. After the first 24−48 hours on 60−80 ml/kg, the fluid intake will need to be adjusted after assessing the infant's clinical appearance, weighing him once or twice daily, and noting his urinary output and plasma electrolytes. The volume required may vary between 20 and 300 ml/kg/24 hours, and may need to be assessed more than once in every 24 hours period.

Electrolyte balance

Problems with electrolyte balance are common in sick neonates, because their kidneys are poor at coping with either too much or too little sodium or potassium.

As with water balance, electrolyte balance problems are rare in infants of any age taking milk orally, except for the hyponatraemia of breast-fed preterm infants (p.107).

Sodium

The normal fullterm infant requires 2−3 mmol/kg/24 hours of sodium. However, the premature kidney may leak 3−5 times more sodium in a given volume of urine than the term kidney, so that sick preterm infants may require up to 15 mmol/kg/24 hours.

Hyponatraemia is common, and is found:

1 In small preterm infants with poor renal sodium conservation.
2 In infants on a low sodium intake (e.g. just EBM, or 10% dextrose).
3 After i.v. frusemide.
4 Following excessive i.v. hypotonic fluid to the mother during labour.
5 In CNS injury due to inappropriate ADH production.

The neonatal kidney has problems in responding to a high plasma sodium with the result that hypernatraemia is found in the following:

1 Small premature infants under radiant heaters which cause marked evaporative water loss and haemoconcentration.
2 Phototherapy, which has a similar effect to radiant heaters and also causes diarrhoea (p.262).
3 Small premature infants receiving i.v. 10% dextrose, causing hyperglycaemia, glycosuria and an osmotic diuresis.
4 Infants who have received too much i.v. sodium bicarbonate.
5 Dehydration from any cause leading to haemoconcentration.

Hyponatraemic infants become listless, develop an ileus and may become hypotensive and convulse. With hypernatraemia, the major hazard is CNS damage and haemorrhage.

Potassium

The neonate needs 2−3 mmol/kg/24 hours of potassium, but this may vary in sick infants.

Hypokalaemia in the neonate usually means overhydration, diuretic use, or that potassium has not been added to an i.v. infusion. Hyperkalemia is usually a sign either of severe illness with potassium leaking out of damaged cells, or of renal failure. Symptoms from hypokalaemia are rare, but hyperkalaemia may cause ventricular tachyarrhythmia and death.

Clinical problems

It is impossible to give a standard sodium and potassium requirement for i.v. therapy in the sick neonate. All sick neonates must have sodium and potassium estimations at least once a day during their period in intensive care. Appropriate adjustments can then be made in their electrolyte intake.

Calcium and phosphate

Calcium and phosphate levels are higher in cord blood than in maternal plasma. Calcium is actively transported from the mother to the fetus and the fetal phosphate rises due to the hypoparathyroidism induced by the relative hypercalcaemia. Postnatally the plasma phosphate may rise due to the low GFR, the relative parathormone deficiency, and a poor phosphaturic response by the kidney to parathormone. Some degree of hypocalcaemia is likely therefore in the neonatal period with values falling to 1.75 mmol/l or less.

Low calcium levels are particularly common:
1 During the first 24−48 hours in any severely ill infant for the above reasons, and also because they have high circulating levels of glucocorticoids and calcitonin and may receive sodium bicarbonate, all of which depress the plasma calcium.
2 In infants of diabetic mothers for similar reasons.
3 During an exchange transfusion with ACD or CPD blood when the citrate in the bank blood chelates the infant's plasma calcium.
Other rare causes of neonatal hypocalcaemia are:
1 Drinking a high phosphate milk (e.g. unadulterated cow's milk): formerly common, now very rare.
2 Renal failure.
3 Primary hypoparathyroidism.
4 Magnesium dependent hypocalcaemia.
5 Di George's syndrome.
6 Maternal hypercalcaemia (e.g. from hyperparathyroidism) causing prolonged neonatal parathyroid depression.
7 Maternal and fetal hypovitaminosis D.

Symptoms

In hypocalcaemic infants less than 72 hours old, convulsions are rare, but heart failure and apnoea may occur; infants on IPPV may become very irritable and jittery. Hypocalcaemia developing during an exchange transfusion may cause convulsions, cardiac arrhythmias or tetany with a positive Chovstek sign. Late onset hypocalcaemia presents with multifocal clonic fits (p.210).

Treatment

In early hypocalcaemia give 5−10 ml of 10% calcium gluconate (1.125−2.25 mmol of calcium^{++})/24 hours orally or i.v. This usually corrects the serum calcium within 24 hours−48 hours and can then be stopped. For tetany, or cardiac arrhythmia during exchange transfusion give 1 ml of 10% calcium gluconate (equivalent to 0.225 mmolCa^{++}) over 2 minutes under ECG control. In late onset hypocalcaemia correction of the underlying problem plus oral calcium supplements are usually effective. Treatment with vitamin D is rarely necessary.

Neonatal hypercalcaemia is rare and usually iatrogenic. Rare cases of neonatal hyperparathyroidism have been described. Hypophosphataemia is rare and usually due to giving intravenous amino-acids without an appropriate phosphate supplement, or long-term feeding of VLBW infants with low phosphate bank breast milk.

Acid base balance

Metabolic acidaemia

All newborn infants have a tendency to metabolic acidaemia due to:
1 The lactic acidaemia following delivery which is more severe if there has been intrapartum asphyxia or severe neonatal respiratory illness.
2 The hydrogen ion load from high solute milks.
3 The hydrogen ion released during normal growth and bone accretion.
4 Their low renal bicarbonate threshold. This is usually 21−22 mmol/l at term, but may be as low as 12 mmol/l in premature infants; although this gives them a low plasma bicarbonate it is not, of course, evidence for a serious illness causing systemic acidosis.
5 The neonatal kidney being poor at excreting hydrogen ions particularly if the baby is ill and preterm. However, even preterm infants increase their ability to excrete hydrogen ions during the first week or two.

The causes of metabolic acidaemia and their management are discussed elsewhere under birth asphyxia (pp.118−19), respiratory disease (p.139), sepsis (p.176), brain disease (p.217), infant feeding (p.109) and inborn errors of metabolism (p.276).

Treatment

Whenever a metabolic acidaemia develops it is essential to establish a cause such as hypotension, hypoxia or sepsis. If these are prevented or quickly recognized and treated, the need to correct metabolic acidaemia will rarely arise. Furthermore it is not usually necessary to correct metabolic acidaemia unless the base deficit exceeds 10 mmol/l (negative base excess of > 10 mmol/l) In chronic situations where the acidaemia is due to a feeding acidosis (p.109) or renal failure it can be corrected by adding sodium bicarbonate to the milk. In emergency situations such as immediately after an asphyxial delivery or cardiorespiratory collapse, where urgent correction is necessary, the dose of bicarbonate is worked out from the equation:
base deficit (mmol/l) × body weight (kg) × 0.3 = dose (in mmol) of bicarbonate.
This should never be infused at a rate exceeding 0.5 mmol/minute.

Metabolic alkalaemia

This is commonly iatrogenic from over-use of bicarbonate, but may be seen after exchange transfusion as the citrate in the blood preservative is metabolized. A compensatory metabolic alkalaemia is seen in infants with chronic lung disease and CO_2 retention.

Respiratory acidaemia

By definition this is a raised P_aCO_2. It is very common in all the respiratory illnessess described in Chapter 15. If mild (up to 8 kPa), and if the infant is otherwise stable, no treatment is required. If higher values occur, IPPV may be necessary.

Respiratory alkalaemia

Many normal newborn babies have a P_aCO_2 of 4.0−4.5 kPa for reasons that are not entirely clear. Levels lower than 4.0 kPa in spontaneously breathing neonates suggest pathological hyperventilation driven either by CNS injury or severe metabolic acidaemia. It is also seen with inappropriately vigorous IPPV.

Chapter 20
Feeding the Sick Neonate

The subject of infant feeding is covered in detail in Chapters 8 and 13. This chapter will concentrate on the nutritional management of ill infants, VLBW babies, and those who are being ventilated.

The following generalizations can be made about feeding sick LBW infants:

1 Infants <32 weeks gestation have enough calorie reserves to survive for only 4−5 days after delivery unless additional calories are given.

2 An adequate fluid and caloric intake are important in preventing early jaundice and hypoglycaemia, both of which can have serious neurological sequelae.

3 After being maintained on i.v. glucose electrolyte solutions for 3−4 days, LBW infants who still do not tolerate oral feeds, or in whom these are still contra-indicated, should be started on intravenous feeding.

4 If very small babies on IPPV for RDS are underfed, they may become so puny and malnourished that they are unable to sustain sufficient power in their respiratory muscles to enable them to be weaned off the ventilator.

5 Although babies on long-term IPPV can be fed enterally, always stop this for 12−24 hours after they are extubated.

6 Infants with septicaemia, severe birth asphyxia, RDS or other serious illnessess virtually always have an ileus during the acute phase of their illness, so that enteral feeding is a complete waste of time.

7 Feeding milk can undoubtedly cause problems (Table 20.1), particularly in VLBW infants. Necrotizing enterocolitis (p.249) may be triggered by using milk-feeding too early.

Feeding routines

Feeding can be started in healthy babies weighing less than 1.5 kg by 3−4 hours of age (Chapter 13).

Ill babies usually lose their ileus by the second to fifth day of their illness, and will then tolerate hourly enteral feeds. In such infants the indications for making an attempt to start enteral feeding are:

1 Absence of abdominal distension.

Table 20.1. Deleterious effects of feeding.

Milk regurgitation and aspiration pneumonia
Recurrent apnoea
Nasal obstruction (*naso*gastric tube only)
Altered respiratory function ($\downarrow P_{a}o_2$, $\downarrow$ FRC)
Introduction of infection (nasogastric or nasojejunal tube)
Necrotizing enterocolitis
Electrolyte imbalance on bank breast milk ($\downarrow$ Na, $\downarrow$ PO$_4$, rickets)
Milk bolus obstruction (rare)
Predisposition to allergy (except breast milk)

2 Meconium passed.
3 Bowel sounds present.
The schedule laid out in Table 13.2 is preferable when starting to feed convalescent VLBW infants, taking day 1 as the first day on which feeding is attempted. In practice, what happens is that a baby starts on 0.5 – 1.0 ml/hour of milk, and this is increased by 0.5 ml every 4 – 6 hours until the correct volumes are achieved.

When starting enteral feeding in sick babies it is absolutely essential to aspirate the baby's nasogastric tube every 4 hours to ensure that the feeds are not pooling in his stomach. If most of the milk given is accumulating, the enteral feeding should be abandoned, and attempted the next day, again starting with 0.5 – 1.0 ml/hour.

Routes of feeding

Giving milk through an indwelling nasogastric tube is the basic technique for feeding all sick babies, using continuous infusion if necessary (Chapter 13).

For the small number of infants who have milk pooling in their stomach, or have problems with regurgitation or apnoea in association with feeding, giving nasojejunal feeds (p.105) may be successful.

What to feed

The ideal milk is EBM from the baby's own mother, and this should always be used if available. Milk from milk banks is deficient in several nutrients and minerals, and if 'mother's-own' is not available, it is preferable to give LBW babies one of the special preterm formulae (p.106).

Intravenous feeding

For the few infants in whom the above ruses fail to provide adequate nourishment, intravenous nutrition is indicated. Initially, this usually takes the form of supplemental nutrition giving glucose/amino-acid/ mineral/vitamin solutions to supplement the small, but inadequate, intakes of milk which are often being tolerated. *Total* parenteral nutrition, using intravenous fat as well, is indicated in the following situations:

1 Neonatal gut malformations — before, during and after surgery.
2 Necrotizing enterocolitis.
3 The occasional baby with serious illness who is unable to tolerate any enteral feeding.

Intravenous feeding, particularly total parenteral nutrition, should not be undertaken lightly in LBW infants, and should only be done in units with adequate medical, nursing, pharmacy and laboratory services.

Contraindications to i.v. feeding

The technique should not be used in infants who:
• Are acidotic (pH < 7.25)
• Have liver damage or are jaundiced
• Are thrombocytopenic

Route of infusion

Intravenous feeding can be given through a peripheral vein. However, the fluids are very irritant, and frequently thrombose the vessels. If extravasation occurs, permanent unpleasant scarring may result. Thus, this route has limited applications and should only be used for i.v. feeding lasting less than a week.

For long-term i.v. feeding it is preferable to use a long line inserted through a peripheral vein and pushed in until the tip lies in a major central vessel. Because of the risk of introducing infection through such a line it should never be used for anything other than the intravenous feeding solution.

Composition of i.v. feeding solution

A solution of 7% vamin in glucose 1890 kJ (450 kCal/l) is the most common solution used for neonates. It should be started at half the maintenance requirement, then built up to a maximum of 42−50 ml/kg/24 hours (equivalent to 3–3.5 g protein/kg/24 hours). Extra glucose can be added to give a final glucose concentration of 12.5–15%. Intralipid 20% (8400 kJ/l [2000 kcal/l]) can be given at 10–15 ml/kg/24 hours, but reduced if lipaemia (triglycerides >2.5 mmol/l [250 mg/100 ml]) develops. The glucose/vamin/electrolyte solution is combined in one infusate and given continuously; the intralipid is also infused continuously through a side arm of the giving set near to the patient. The electrolyte content, including Ca^{++} and PO_4''' can be varied daily depending on the baby's needs.

Multivitamin preparations are given once daily; folic acid, vitamins B_{12}, D and K and trace metals need to be given if *total* parenteral nutrition is given for more than a week.

Complications of i.v. feeding

These come under four main headings:

Catheter-related. If the solutions infused through a central catheter are heparinized then this virtually eliminates thrombotic complications; haemorrhage from these narrow bore tubes is unlikely.

Infection. This is a major problem with central lines. Infants should have blood cultures weekly or if pyrexia develops. If infection is confirmed or if pyrexia persists despite negative cultures, remove the line.

Metabolic. By rigorous attention to the details of the electrolyte, glucose and vitamin infusion, and appropriate adjustments of the rate of infusion, these can be more or less eliminated.

Jaundice. In premature infants cholestatic jaundice develops after 2–3 weeks of intravenous feeding. The mechanism is not understood. If possible, the i.v. feeding should be discontinued.

Chapter 21
Gastroenterological Problems in the Newborn

Congenital malformations

Tracheo-oesophageal fistula (oesophageal atresia)
(incidence 1:3500)

85% of cases have an upper oesophageal atresia, with a fistula from the carina to the lower oesphagus. 7% have oesophageal atresia with a blind ending lower oesophagus but no tracheal connection.

Diagnosis

The mother usually has hydramnios; after delivery the baby chokes and splutters on his secretions which he cannot swallow. These may be inhaled, causing an aspiration pneumonia.

The diagnosis is confirmed by failing to pass a wide bore (FG 10–12) oro-gastric tube. A plain X-ray of the chest and abdomen with this tube *in situ* will confirm that it is stuck in the oesophagus at the level of T2–T4, and will also show whether gas is present in the bowel. If present, this confirms the existence of a tracheo-oesophageal fistula and suggests that the infant has the common type of malformation. If there is no gas in the bowel, then a fistula is absent. Contrast studies to confirm oesophageal atresia are not necessary.

Management

Total surgical correction should be undertaken as soon as possible in babies with the common variant, but with rarer forms it may be necessary to do a oesophagostomy and gastrostomy, and reconstruct the oesphagus later in life.

Pre-operatively, prevent inhalation pneumonia by regularly aspirating a tube in the oesophageal pouch; keep the baby head-up to prevent reflux through the fistula.

Post-operatively, once bowel sounds return, feed the infant through the trans-anastomotic nasogastric tube which will have been left in position at operation.

Diaphagmatic hernia (incidence 1:4000)

90% are left-sided through the foramen of Bochdalek, the rest being right-sided, or herniae through the retrosternal foramina of Morgani.

Two-thirds of cases have severe pulmonary hypoplasia which is incompatible with life even if the diaphragmatic defect is rapidly repaired.

Diagnosis

Most babies present at birth when, due to pulmonary hypoplasia, resuscitation is very difficult. Characteristically, they have a scaphoid abdomen since the abdominal contents are lying in the chest. Despite high pressure IPPV, they remain difficult to oxygenate. Small herniae may present during the first few days of life with dyspnoea and bowel sounds in the chest.

The diagnosis is confirmed by demonstrating intrathoracic bowel shadows on chest X-ray.

Treatment

The diaphragmatic defect should be repaired as soon after diagnosis as possible, though the pulmonary hypoplasia may be so severe that the infant never gets to the theatre. In others the hypoplasia causes irremediable post-operative respiratory failure.

In infants who are easy to oxygenate pre-operatively the post-operative recovery is usually smooth, though they may have a period with PFC (p.201).

Gut malformations presenting with intestinal obstruction

Intestinal obstruction with abdominal distention, constipation, pooling of gastric contents and bile-stained aspirates is common in preterm babies with an ileus due to RDS, septicaemia or NEC. These conditions are easily recognized (Table 21.1), and in an otherwise well baby with intestinal obstruction, structural malformation of the bowel is very likely.

Duodenal atresia (incidence 1:6000)

33% of cases have Down's syndrome, and about 50% of chromosomally normal infants with duodenal atresia have other malformations.

Table 21.1. Differential diagnosis of abdominal distention and bilious vomiting in the neonate.

Condition	Evaluation and differential diagnosis
Necrotizing enterocolitis (p.249)	Generally septic picture and blood in stools; abdominal X-ray: fluid levels and gas in bowel wall; ascites
Paralytic ileus	Any very sick infant, e.g. RDS, sepsis
Small intestinal atresia including post ampullary duodenal atresia, and volvulus with malrotation	Infant otherwise well. Plain X-ray; fluid levels, though infant may have passed meconium. Barium meal shows duodenum in wrong place with malrotation
Meconium ileus	Family history of cystic fibrosis; peculiar bubbly gut contents on abdominal X-ray; Infants rarely pass meconium
Large bowel obstruction (Hirschsprung's or meconium plug)	Usually no meconium passed. No gas in rectum. Barium enema usually diagnostic (and sometimes therapeutic)
Imperforate anus	Obvious! (hopefully)

Duodenal atresia presents in the first 24 hours of life with vomiting, which may not be bilious since the obstruction can occur proximal to the ampulla of Vater. Meconium may be passed, since the lower bowel is normal. The diagnosis is confirmed by the classical double bubble appearance on the erect abdominal X-ray (Fig. 21.1).

Although rarer malformations like annular pancreas or peritoneal (Ladd's) bands can give a similar clinical and X-ray picture, these can only be differentiated at laparotomy, which should be carried out as soon as possible.

Small intestinal obstruction

This can be caused by atresia or malrotation. Atresias present within 48 hours of birth with abdominal distention and bilious vomiting, but a malrotation may not develop a volvulus and obstruct until much later in life, and only about 50% will present in the neonatal period. In both conditions the baby may pass meconium.

Diagnosis

An erect abdominal X-ray shows fluid levels in the absence of other causes of obstruction such as NEC (Table 21.1).

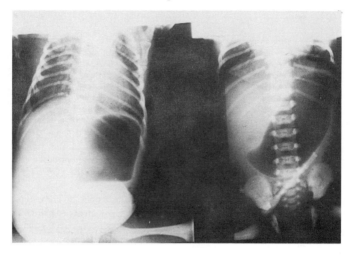

Fig. 21.1. Double bubble in duodenal atresia. Erect picture on left, supine on right.

A barium meal will identify a malrotation by the abnormal position of the duodenum and will do no harm in infants with other causes of obstruction.

Treatment

All cases require laparotomy and it should be carried out as soon as possible to prevent necrosis of the gut involved in the volvulus.

Meconium ileus

This neonatal manifestation of cystic fibrosis is due to obstruction of the small intestine by extremely viscid meconium. About 10% of patients with cystic fibrosis present this way. Prenatally it may cause intra-uterine bowel perforation, and meconium peritonitis.

The baby has bilious vomiting and marked abdominal distention from birth. The following clues help to differentiate it from other causes of neonatal obstruction:
1 Meconium is not passed.
2 A family history of cystic fibrosis.
3 Abdominal X-rays show a foamy appearance of gut contents.
4 With meconium peritonitis flecks of intra-abdominal calcification are seen.

Diagnosis

Do a gastrografin enema using up to 100 ml of undiluted contrast. By using this intensely hydrophilic material not only can other diagnoses be excluded, but since the gastrografin draws fluid into the gut, it liquifies the very stickly meconium, which may then be passed. Several enemata may be given, but if they do not relieve the obstruction, laparotomy is necessary to empty the tacky meconium out of the terminal ileum.

Hirschsprung's disease (incidence 1:5000)

This is the congenital absence of Meissner's and Auerbach's plexuses extending proximally from the internal anal sphincter. Although even small bowel can be involved, the aganglionic segment rarely extends proximal to the sigmoid colon. Skip lesions do not occur.

Hirschsprung's usually presents by 48–72 hours of age with abdominal distension, bilious vomiting and complete constipation. A rectal examination reveals a small rectum and is often followed by the explosive passage of flatus and faeces. Otherwise normal neonates who have not passed meconium by 48 hours should be suspected of Hirschsprung's disease.

Diagnosis

A plain abdominal X-ray shows distended bowel loops but fluid levels are comparatively sparse, which helps differentiate Hirschsprung's disease from small intestinal obstruction. A barium enema should be done to support the diagnosis but also to exclude other conditions (Table 21.1). The diagnosis is confirmed by suction biopsy of the rectal mucosa.

Do not do a rectal wash-out before the enema, since this changes the characteristic X-ray appearance in Hirschsprung's which is a coned transition zone where the dilated normal bowel reaches the narrow aganglionic segment.

Treatment

A defunctioning colostomy should be formed proximal to the obstruction. Excision of the involved segment and the pull-through operation bringing normal bowel to the anus should be deferred until the infant is 6–12 months old.

Meconium plug

This presents like Hirschsprung's disease, but following rectal examination, or a diagnostic enema, the plug is passed. The condition may coexist with other forms of bowel disease such as meconium ileus or Hirschsprung's, and these diagnoses should be considered if bowel function does not become normal immediately after passing the plug.

Imperforate anus/rectal agenesis (incidence 1:5000)

The rectum may terminate anywhere from above the levator ani down to the anus, which may be covered by nothing more than a thin membrane through which meconium can be seen.

Diagnosis

This is obvious, but to assess the level of the obstruction, the baby should have an AP and laternal X-ray of the abdomen and pelvis with the position of his anus marked. Other malformations, including fistulae into the urinary or genital tract are common, and the infants should have appropriate post-operative X-ray investigations.

Treatment

The baby requires a defunctioning colostomy, unless a small incision in an anal membrane will create a patent bowel. Corrective surgery is carried out at 6−12 months.

Gastroschisis

A defect in the abdominal wall above the umbilicus through which gut contents, not covered by peritonium, herniate (incidence 1:30 000).

Exomphalos (omphalocele).

A herniation through the umbilical hiatus of gut contents covered by peritonium (incidence 1:2500).

In exomphalos, there is a high incidence of other lethal malformations, and malrotation commonly coexists with gastroschisis.

Treatment

Immediately after birth the exposed bowel should be covered with a plastic bag or a layer of 'clingfilm'. Immediate repair of the defect may be possible in infants with a small exomphalos. If, in either condition, the contents of the hernia are too big to fit into the abdominal cavity, but are forcibly replaced at an initial operation, this causes diaphragmatic splinting, respiratory failure and death. In such cases the exposed bowel should be enclosed in a silastic bag which is stitched to the edge of the defect. Over a period of weeks, the bag is gradually rolled up, slowly returning its contents to a growing abdominal cavity. When everything is replaced, muscle and skin closure can be carried out.

Post-operative care

Post-operative management of these surgical problems is more or less identical and is based on:
1 Careful attention to nursing routines, e.g. hourly turning and oropharyngeal suction.
2 Daily PCV and electrolyte measurements, with appropriate adjustment in i.v. fluids and blood transfusion.
3 Regular blood gas analysis.
4 Continuous ECG monitoring.
5 IPPV if necessary.
6 Antibiotics. Most surgeons prefer these infants to have post-operative antibiotics. Use the cocktail in current use in the unit (p.176).
7 Total parenteral nutrition, in most cases for 5−10 days.

Necrotizing enterocolitis

This disease usually affects the terminal ileum and the colon, and is most common in ill premature infants. However, individual cases and epidemics occur in previously well fullterm babies.

Aetiology (Fig. 21.2)

Many factors diminish mucosal blood flow. In addition, invasion of the ischaemic mucosa by gas-forming organisms from the gut is necessary. NEC is more common in fluid-overloaded babies and virtually never happens until the neonate has had milk.

Symptoms and signs

In mild cases the infant may show early signs of infection (pp.172−4)

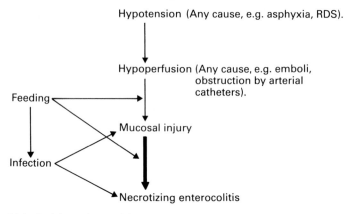

Fig. 21.2. Aetiology of necrotizing enterocolitis.

and often passes bloody stools. As the disease progresses the infant looks iller, abdominal distention increases and the stools are more bloody. Eventually the infant becomes obstructed and has an ileus, with absent bowel sounds and bilious or faeculent vomiting. The distended abdomen may be tender, with induration of the abdominal wall over areas of involved gut.

Diagnosis

Do the usual tests carried out to exclude infection (p.175); X-raying the abdomen establishes diagnosis. In mild cases there may be occasional fluid levels, and the gut wall seems thicker than usual. In more severe cases gas bubbles are seen initially in the bowel wall and eventually in the liver within the biliary tree. Ascites may be present, and if intestinal perforation occurs free gas will be seen. Barium studies are not necessary.

Differential diagnosis

The history, clinical examination and X-ray findings are characteristic (Table 21.1) A pneumoperitoneum may occur during high pressure IPPV, (p.151) and is usually easy to differentiate. Bleeding rectally from local causes such as fissure-in-ano must be excluded (p.252).

Treatment

Stop oral feeding, and start a 'drip and suck' regime. Maintain hydration and nutrition intravenously, giving full TPN (p.241). Correct hypotension, anaemia, acidaemia and respiratory failure. The infants lose a large amount of protein-rich fluid as ascites, and frequent blood and/or plasma transfusion are important.

The usual antibiotic cocktail (p.176) should be given intravenously, plus metronidazole in view of the importance of anaerobic organisms in gut infections. This conservative management should be continued for 7–10 days with abdominal X-rays taken at least daily to detect bowel perforation as soon as possible. If this occurs, laparotomy should be carried out with resection of involved segments of gut.

Laparotomy should also be considered in cases who show no response to conservative treatment, and in whom an ileus with ascites persists for more than 4–5 days.

Sequelae

The mortality is 20–30% amongst infants who perforate, but should be less than 10% in those who do not. About 10% of infants develop a further typical attack of NEC. In 5–10% of those who did not need laparotomy the affected bit of gut stenoses. This presents later with signs of intestinal obstruction, though the baby is otherwise healthy. This stenosed segment should be excised.

Diarrhoea and vomiting in the neonate

If both of these are present the diagnosis is usually gastro-enteritis (p.181).

Vomiting

Many newborn babies vomit immediately after delivery: this is usually ascribed to swallowed blood, mucus or meconium, and stops following a stomach wash-out. Other neonates may vomit intermittently for several days before they gradually settle down, and no cause is ever found for this symptom. However, persistent vomiting, particularly if it becomes bilious or faeculent, is usually due to intestinal obstruction (p.244). In infants who are overtly ill and vomiting copiously, it is important not to forget three rarities which can present in the neonatal period, and which are important to detect and treat early:
● Galactosaemia (p.275)
● Congenital adrenal hyperplasia (p.273)
● Hyperammonaemia (p.276)

The common causes of vomiting in older infants can occasionally present later in the neonatal period. These include:

- Upper respiratory tract infections
- Otitis media
- Infection — urinary, meningitis, etc.
- Pyloric stenosis
- Hiatus hernia

If vomiting is peristent in the absence of clinical findings it may occasionally be necessary to carry out a barium meal to exclude rare causes of sub-acute intestinal obstruction.

Diarrhoea

Persisting diarrhoea is very rare in the newborn. If diarrhoea with weight-loss or dehydration presents in the absence of gastro-enteritis, sugar intolerance should be considered if there is at least 1% sugar in the stools tested by the 'Clinitest' method. There are three possible diagnoses:

1 Post gastro-enteritis sugar intolerance.
2 Post neonatal surgery sugar intolerance.
3 Congenital defects in brush border enzymes.

The first two conditions are readily diagnosed by exclusion, and treatment is to remove lactose from the diet for several weeks. Occasionally it is also necessary to withdraw cow's milk protein, or even resort to i.v. feeding until the bowel recovers.

Diarrhoea due to congenital defects in bowel function is exceptionally rare, but should be considered if intractable diarrhoea persists.

Haematemesis, melaena and bloody stools in the newborn

Minor degrees of these are very common, and the following conditions should be excluded before indulging in complex X-ray studies or investigating the clotting mechanism:

- Swallowed maternal/placental blood at delivery
- Swallowed maternal blood from a cracked nipple
- Local trauma, e.g. from a nasogastric tube, following laryngoscopy or over-vigorous laryngeal suction
- Fissure-in-ano

Always check whether such blood is maternal (swallowed) or fetal by using Apt's test for fetal haemoglobin. When 1% NaOH is added to a dilute solution of the bloody effluent in water, fetal haemoglobin stays pink, whereas adult haemoglobin denatures and goes brown. The serious causes of haematemesis or blood in the stools are:

• Necrotizing enterocolitis (p.249)
• Haemorrhagic diatheses of various types including haemorrhagic disease of the newborn and DIC (p.291)
• Rare problems:
  trauma (e.g. broken rectal thermometer)
  Meckel's diverticulum
  malrotation
  peptic ulceration
  rectal polyps/haemangiomas
  colitis
  intussusception
  gut reduplication

These should only be sought if the other conditions have been excluded, and bleeding persists.

Chapter 22
Jaundice and Liver Disease

Jaundice in the newborn is important for two reasons:
1 It may indicate severe underlying disease.
2 Unconjugated bilirubin is neurotoxic.

Physiology of bilirubin (Fig. 22.1)

Most bilirubin (75%) is derived from the breakdown of red cells. Each gram of haemoglobin yields 595 μmol of bilirubin in the unconjugated 'indirect' form, most of which is tightly bound to albumin and is water insoluble, only nanomole quantities are unbound. In the liver conjugation occurs in the smooth endoplasmic reticulum, catalysed by glucuronyl transferase. The resulting water soluble bilirubin diglucuronide (conjugated or 'direct' bilirubin) is excreted via the bile ducts into the intestine.

Normally, urine contains no bile, but if hepatic excretion is obstructed, conjugated bilirubin is 'regurgitated' into the circulation and excreted by the kidney.

Fetal and neonatal bilirubin metabolism

Fetal bilirubin is cleared across the placenta and processed by the maternal liver. If there is excessive haemolysis some unconjugated bilirubin appears in the amniotic fluid; the mechanism for this is uncertain.

Red cell turnover in the fetus and neonate is high compared with that in adults because:
1 Red cell mass (40 ml/kg) is relatively large.
2 Fetal red cells have a shorter life span (40−60 versus 120 days).

As a result 135−170 μmol bilirubin/kg/day is generated — twice the adult production; conjugation of this in the neonate is limited by a relative lack of glucuronyl transferase, more marked in premature infants.

The meconium in the gut of the neonate contains about 200 mg (3400 μmol) of conjugated bilirubin. An enzyme in the gut (beta glucuronidase) hydrolyzes conjugated bilirubin, the unconjugated

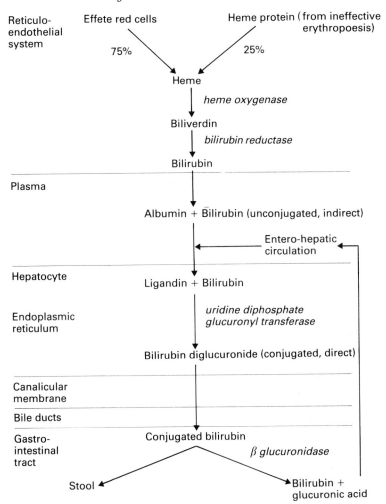

Fig. 22.1. Metabolism of bilirubin.

form is then reabsorbed via the entero-hepatic circulation; this reaction may be an important contributor to jaundice when there is intestinal stasis (ileus, delayed passage of meconium).

In the first few days, for all these reasons bilirubin production may surpass excretory capacity and the *unconjugated* bilirubin may rise to potentially toxic levels. *Conjugated* hyperbilirubinaemia only occurs if there is hepato-cellular damage or a block in the biliary tree; it is rare in the neonate. Conjugated bilirubin is not toxic.

Bilirubin neurotoxicity (kernicterus)

In the past high bilirubin levels, in particular when caused by haemolytic disease of the newborn (HDN), were associated with often fatal neonatal neurological disease with yellow stained basal nuclei seen at necropsy (kernicterus). Since then many follow-up studies have shown an association between high neonatal bilirubin levels and subsequent athetoid cerebral palsy. Deafness can also occur and may be a sequel of much lower bilirubin levels in preterm infants.

Pathophysiology

Bilirubin, when bound to membranes, is cytotoxic, but why it binds to them is still unclear. Probably what matters is the relative binding affinity of bilirubin with either albumin or cell membranes and the amount of unbound bilirubin in plasma and brain ECF. The normal neonatal blood brain barrier is probably permeable to free bilirubin but is impermeable to protein. It will open, however, under the influence of hypoxia/ischaemia when albumin-bound bilirubin as well as unbound bilirubin can then cross. In the brain ECF, acidosis favours the binding of bilirubin to cells, whereas at normal pH albumin binding would be favoured.

Factors influencing the development of kernicterus, therefore, are:

1 Low serum albumin: by reducing the bilirubin binding capacity and increasing the amount of unbound bilirubin.

2 Displacement of bilirubin from albumin binding sites by

  a Excess free fatty acids which may be elevated in:
- Hypoxia/ischaemia
- Hypoglycaemia
- Infection
- Starvation
- Administration of intralipid

  b Drugs: although this has been shown *in vitro* for many drugs, only sufisoxazole has been shown to increase the risk of kernicterus *in vivo*.

3 Hypoxia/ischaemia: by opening the blood brain barrier.

4 Acidaemia: by favouring tissue binding of bilirubin.

None of the laboratory methods used to assess these interactions have proved reliable, so that the total serum bilirubin and the clinical state of the infant are still the only guides to the risk of kernicterus at a given bilirubin level in an individual baby. As a result no safe level of bilirubin has been established, but the levels of bilirubin at which therapy is recommended are given in Table 22.1.

Table 22.1 Guidelines for treating unconjugated hyperbilirubinaemia with phototherapy and exchange transfusion.

Bilirubin (mmol/l)	Birthweight (g)				
	<1000	1000−1500	1500−2000	2000−2500	>2500
100	PT	OR	O	O	O
150		PT	OR	O	O
200	XT		PT	OR	O
250		XT		PT	OR
300			XT		PT
350				XT	
400					XT

O = observe, OR = observe and repeat bilirubin, PT = phototherapy, XT = exchange transfusion.

Notes
1 The respective levels for phototherapy and exchange transfusion should be lowered by at least one stage if the infant is ill, acidotic, hypoglycaemic, or hypoalbuminaemic.
2 These guidelines do not apply to infants with rhesus HDN (p.264).

Early onset unconjugated jaundice (see Table 22.2)

Aetiology

Physiological

A combination of factors, one of which may predominate, leads to so-called physiological jaundice.
1 Increased bilirubin load secondary to:
   a Polycythaemia (p.289).
   b Decreased red cell cell survival (see above).
   c Extravasated blood (bruising, cephalhaematoma)
2 Relative deficiency of glucuronyl transferase.
3 Increased entero-hepatic circulation secondary to:
   a Delayed enteral feeding and meconium passage.
   b Intestinal obstruction.
   c Swallowed blood.
4 Breast-feeding due to low fluid and calorie intake.

Table 22.2. Differential diagnosis of jaundice appearing in the first 5 days (unconjugated hyperbilirubinaemia).

Age	Cause	Features	Tests
1–2 days	Haemolytic disease Rh (D)	Usually known antenatally, may be no clinical signs, or pallor + hepatosplenomegaly	Do blood group, Coombs' test, Hb, PCV on all suspected haemolytic disease (Rh or ABO)
	Other Rh (C, c, E, e)	As above	Look for maternal antibodies
	ABO	Usually not known antenatally, Anaemia and hepatospenomegaly rare	Mother group O, baby group A or B Look for maternal haemolysins
	Congenital spherocytosis	Positive family history	Blood film
	Congenital infection (very rare)	SFD, hepatosplenomegaly, petechiae	Platelet count, IgM, serology, appropriate viral cultures
>2 days	Physiological (very common)	Well baby, no other signs	Measure bilirubin as necessary
	Late onset HDN (particularly ABO)	As above	As above
	Bacterial sepsis	Lethargy, fever, vomiting, abdominal distension (p.174)	Blood count, culture blood, urine, CSF, superficial swabs as above
	Congenital infection	As above	
	Abnormal red cell morphology Congenital spherocytosis Elliptocytosis	Positive family history (autosomal dominant) (autosomal dominant)	Blood count and blood film
	Red cell enzyme defects G6PD deficiency	Ethnic group-Mediterranean, Oriental, African. X-linked inheritance	G6PD screening test
	Pyruvate kinase deficiency	autosomal recessive inheritance	Red cell pyruvate kinase

Pathological

1 Excessive haemolysis due to:
a Blood group incompatability (p.264).
b Septicaemia (bacterial haemolysins) (Chapter 16).
c Congenital structural red cell defects (spherocytosis, elliptocytosis) (Chapter 25).
d Inherited red cell enzyme defects (G6PD, pyruvate kinase deficiency) (Chapter 25).
2 Inherited metabolic defects (very rare, usually prolonged, p.263).

Differential diagnosis and investigation (Table 22.2)

The most likely causes can often be inferred from:
1 Time of onset (day 1, days 2–5, >5 days).
2 Maternal and/or family history.
3 Pattern of jaundice (rapid rise, gradual increase, prolonged).
4 Presence of associated signs or symptoms.

Jaundice on the first day

Any jaundice noted within 24 hours *must* be regarded as haemolytic disease until proved otherwise (p.264). The following features suggest that it could be serious:
● Pallor
● Palpable liver and spleen
● Rh negative mother
● Mother blood group O with baby group A or B (p.268)
● Family history of spherocytosis or splenectomy
● Anything suggesting congenital infection (p.185)

Jaundice noted at 2–5 days

Up to 50% of normal-term infants develop physiological jaundice, the incidence is much higher in preterm babies; it follows a characteristic pattern with onset after the first 48 hours, reaching a peak on day 3–5, remaining elevated for several days and then gradually declining. In preterm infants the level may remain high for longer.
Before diagnosing 'physiological' jaundice always:
1 Consider the features listed above.
2 Look for precipitating factors for physiological jaundice. Is the baby premature, bruised or very plethoric (do PCV). Is the mother diabetic (p.289)?
3 Think of infection. If in any doubt, investigate (p.175, Table 22.2).

Bilirubin measurements

Jaundice becomes clinically evident at bilirubin levels of 80−120 μmol/l. Many term infants become slightly yellow (<170 μmol/l) after 48 hours and it is unnecessary to measure their bilirubin provided they are clinically well. It takes a little practice to distinguish mild jaundice (<170 μmol/l) from levels that are potentially serious and the neophyte neonatologist will initially measure many more bilirubins than necessary.

Clinical estimations are notoriously difficult in:
• Artificial light
• Coloured infants (look at the conjunctivae)

Always measure bilirubin if:
1 *Any* degree of jaundice is noted on the first day.
2 There are known maternal antibodies.
3 Gestation <35 weeks or birthweight <2000 g.
4 The infant is unwell in any way.
5 There is hepato-splenomegaly, petechiae or CNS disturbance.
6 Onset >4 days.
7 Prolonged jaundice (>12−14 days).

Prolonged unconjugated jaundice

Jaundice persisting for more than 14 days requires investigation. It is important to exclude *conjugated* hyperbilirubinaemia (which, if present, is investigated as outlined on p.263).

Aetiology of prolonged unconjugated jaundice

1 Prolonged physiological jaundice, particularly in premature infants.
2 Persistent haemolytic jaundice:
 a Immune.
 b Congenital spherocytosis.
 c Red cell enzyme defects.
3 Chronic sepsis.
4 Breast milk jaundice.
5 Hypothyroidism.
6 Galactosaemia (often a conjugated hyperbilirubinaemia, p.275).
7 Cystic fibrosis.
8 Rare inherited disorders of bilirubin metabolism:
 a Crigler−Najjar syndromes.
 b Gilbert's disease.
 c Lucey−Driscoll syndrome.

Breast milk jaundice

This is the commonest cause of prolonged unconjugated jaundice in healthy infants and occurs in 0.5−2.5% of those who are breast-fed; to some extent it is a diagonsis of exclusion. Characteristically the bilirubin reaches a peak at 10−15 days, persists for 4−10 days and then gradually declines over 3−12 weeks. The following aetiological theories have been proposed but none are proven.

1 High lipoprotein lipase content in breast milk liberating large amounts of free fatty acids which inhibit bilirubin conjugation.

2 The presence of a steroid (3α-20β pregnanediol) which inhibits conjugation from the gut.

3 Increased enterohepatic circulation due to some factor in breast milk which promotes bilirubin reabsorption from the gut.

Management

Breast milk jaundice is not dangerous and always resolves spontaneously; exclude serious conditions. Although stopping breast-feeding will cause the bilirubin to fall, this is not indicated.

Diagnostic approach to prolonged jaundice
not due to breast milk (see Table 22.2 for investigations)

Exclude persistent haemolytic syndromes and sepsis.
Think of hypothyroidism and cystic fibrosis (neonatal screening now done, see p.87), and galactosaemia (p.275).
The inherited disorders of bilirubin metabolism are very rare.

Treatment of unconjugated jaundice
(irrespective of cause)

This varies with gestational age: the more immature the infant the more aggressive should be the treatment. The following general measures are recommended although the scientific evidence for their efficacy is dubious.

1 Early enteral feeding helps to stimulate peristalsis and clear meconium from the intestine, hence reducing the entero-hepatic circulation.

2 Avoid or treat dehydration. Give an *adequate* fluid intake but there is no evidence that *extra* fluid has any effect in lowering bilirubin.

Phototherapy

Unconjugated bilirubin undergoes a geometric photo-isomerization to forms that can be directly excreted without conjugation. There is no evidence that these 'photobilirubins' are neurotoxic. The effectiveness of phototherapy is measured in units of irradiance at wavelengths 425−475 nm and the minimum required is 4 μW/cm^2.

Indications

1 As an adjunct to management of HDN (p.267).
2 For other unconjugated hyperbilirubinaemias, but the cause should be established first. The bilirubin levels for starting phototherapy are indicated in Table 22.1.

Side effects

1 Although there is no direct evidence in humans of light-induced eye damage, it seems prudent to patch the eyes during phototherapy.
2 Decreased gut transit time with loose green stools and increased fluid loss.
3 Increased evaporative water loss due to overhead heat.
4 Increased stool loss of N, Na$^+$ and K$^+$; thus weight gain may be less.
5 Psychological effect on the mother; the sight of an eye-bandaged baby may be very distressing.
6 'Bronze baby' syndrome. If there is a cholestatic (conjugated) jaundice, brown photo-degradation pigments are formed, giving the baby a bronzed appearance.

Guidelines on the use of phototherapy

• Pay careful attention to fluid and electrolyte balance
• Make serial measurements of bilirubin — clinical judgment of skin colour becomes invalid

Exchange transfusion

This is the technique which must be used when reduction of plasma bilirubin levels is urgent (Table 22.1).
Indications:
• HDN (p.267)
• Septicaemia (p.177)
• Severe physiological jaundice in premature infants (Table 22.1)

Conjugated hyperbilirubinaemia (>75 μmol/l)

A number of conditions are associated with a conjugated hyperbilirubinaemia; laboratory investigation is essential to sort them out. Their onset is usually after 7 days (although it may follow earlier unconjugated jaundice) which may be after the infant has gone home. Hepatomegaly and splenomegaly are frequently present. The urine usually contains bile.

Aetiology

1 'Toxic' hepatitis secondary to:
 a Sepsis (p.174).
 b Parenteral nutrition (p.242).
2 Infectious hepatitis:
 a TORCH infections (p.184) (toxoplasmosis, rubella, cytomegalovirus, herpes).
 b Other viruses. e.g.entero-viruses.
 c Hepatitis A or B.
3 Inherited metabolic disorders:
 a α-1-antitrypsin deficiency.
 b Galactosaemia (p.275).
 c Cystic fibrosis.
4 Inspissated bile syndrome following severe HDN.
5 Biliary atresia.
6 Extrinsic biliary obstruction, e.g. choledochal cyst.
7 Idiopathic giant cell hepatitis

The commonest causes of neonatal cholestatic jaundice are sepsis and that associated with intravenous nutrition. 75% of the remainder are due to idiopathic giant cell hepatitis and biliary atresia, which can be difficult to distinguish on clinical and laboratory grounds alone.

Diagnostic approach

1 Exclude sepsis by blood and urine cultures.
2 Look for other signs of congenital infection and do appropriate serology.
3 Exclude inherited metabolic defects:
 a Galactosaemia (p.275).
 b Blood for α-1-antitrypsin.
 c Sweat test for cystic fibrosis.
  Extrahepatic obstruction can often be diagnosed by ultrasound. Differentiating biliary atresia from idiopathic giant cell hepatitis requires biochemical tests, ultrasound, radioactive tracers, and percu-

taneous liver biopsy, but may only be possible at laparotomy. However, diagnosis must be made promptly since successful operation in
biliary atresia — the Kasai procedure, in which bowel is anastomosed
direct to the porta hepatis, is less likely after 7–8 weeks of age. Giant
cell hepatitis requires no specific therapy and recovery is the rule.

Haemolytic disease of the newborn
(erythroblastosis fetalis)

Rhesus isoimmunization

This results from an immune response by an Rh negative mother to
the red cells of her rhesus (D) positive fetus.

Mechanism

There are small leaks of blood from fetus to mother in all pregnancies,
with large leaks at the time of delivery or abortion (spontaneous or
induced). Leaked rhesus positive (D +ve) fetal red cells can stimulate
an antibody response in a Rh negative mother, especially if fetus and
mother are ABO compatible (if they are incompatible the fetal red
cells are usually destroyed before antibody can be made). A leak of
more than about 1 ml is probably needed to induce a primary antibody response. Leaks of this size occur mainly at the time of delivery
so that only 5% of primiparae are affected by feto-maternal bleeds
occuring earlier in the pregnancy. In the 95% of mothers who only
develop antibodies post partum, the small feto-maternal leaks which
occur during subsequent pregnancies with a D+ve fetus can, however, provoke a major antibody response.

The IgG antibodies cross the placenta and attack the fetal red cells
(haemolytic disease). The fetus responds by a compensatory increase
in erythropoiesis (erythroblastosis). If haemolysis is severe the fetus
becomes severely anaemic and may even go into heart failure (hydrops
fetalis) and die. Severity of disease tends to increase with each affected
pregnancy.

Prevention of HDN

By giving Rh (D) antibody to all Rh negative women within 72 hours
after delivery of a Rh (D) +ve fetus, the leaked fetal red cells are
destroyed before they can elicit any antibody response. Similarly,
anti-D is also given to Rh negative women after any event or proce-

dure capable of promoting a feto-maternal bleed, e.g. abortion, amniocentesis, ectopic pregnancy or external version.

Antenatal detection and management

1 Group all mothers at booking.
2 Group consorts of Rh negative women, if they are Rh negative, there is no risk to the fetus.
3 Screen all Rh negative mothers for antibodies. If found, follow the levels serially (expressed as μg/ml antibody protein); however, these do not accurately reflect severity of the disease.
4 If the antibody level exceeds 1.5 μg/ml in a first affected pregnancy or 1.0 μg/ml in a subsequent one the most accurate test of severity is to examine the amniotic fluid for bilirubin by spectrophotometry.

The normally clear and colourless liquor becomes yellow in the presence of haemolysis. The concentration of bilirubin is too low (<17 μmol/l) to measure by conventional methods. The optical density of normal amniotic fluid, when plotted on a semi-logarithmic scale over the wavelengths 365−550 nm, describes a straight line, but in the presence of bile pigment there is a peak at 450 nm. The optical density difference between this peak and the straight line gives a measure of bilirubin, meconium or blood in the fluid invalidates the results.

The optical density difference is then plotted on a chart relating GA to fetal risk (Fig. 22.2). Values in zone 3 indicate a severely affected fetus in imminent danger of death. Serial analyses provide the best guide to prognosis and management, two or three specimens obtained at 1−2 week intervals being essential to observe the trend. Delivery can be planned on the basis of these results. *Very* occasionally a badly affected, premature fetus needs intra-uterine transfusion.

Delivery

1 On the basis of GA, antibody levels and amniocentesis results, affected infants should be delivered electively (by induction or caesarean section); timing is crucial, the decision being a joint one between obstetrician and paediatrician.
2 Always have fresh rhesus negative blood (cross-matched against the mother) ready for the baby in case early exchange transfusion is needed (p.267).
3 If a premature (<34 weeks) or severely affected infant is expected, two paediatricians should attend for resuscitation.
4 Send cord blood urgently for group, Coombs' test and Hb.

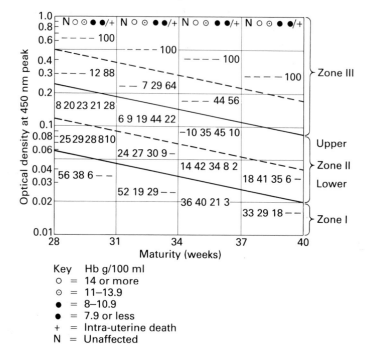

Fig. 22.2. Percentage probability of the various grades of severity for the optical density in a single specimen of liquor. Maturity in brackets of 3 weeks. (Data from Liley, 1963.)

Clinical features and early management

Immediately after delivery and resuscitation note any pallor and hepatosplenomegaly (evidence of extra-medullary haemopoiesis). Remember that the baby may also have RDS. Infants can be broadly separated into groups as follows:

Very severe (hydrops fetalis). Desparately sick, pale+++, oedematous, respiratory distress, ascites, hepato-splenomegaly+++, cord Hb <5 g, bilirubin >85 μmol. These infants are in gross heart failure and need expert intensive care if they are to survive; this includes (p.320):
• IPPV from birth is mandatory
• Draining ascites and pleural effusions
• Immediate exchange transfusion preferably with packed red cells
• Diuretics

Severe. Pale but not hydropic, massive hepato-splenomegaly; cord Hb usually 5−10 g, bilirubin 50−120 μmol. These infants need exchange transfusion within 60−90 minutes with fresh whole blood.

Moderately severe. Pale, hepato-splenomegaly usual, cord Hb 10−12 g, bilirubin <85 μmol. These infants will need exchange within the next 6 hours.

Mild. Not clinically anaemic, hepato-splenomegaly absent or minimal, cord Hb >13 g. One can afford to await developments in these infants; exchange is done on the basis of serial bilirubin measurements (see below).

Subsequent management

1 Measure the bilirubin 6-hourly and plot the results against postnatal age to monitor the rate of rise. Prevent the bilirubin from rising above 340 μmol in term infants, lower in premature ones (Table 22.1).
2 If the rate of rise exceeds 17 μmol/hour, exchange transfusion will certainly be necessary and should be done without waiting for a further rise. This will reduce the bilirubin by about 30−60% but there will be a rebound rise later.
3 Give phototherapy (p.262) if bilirubin >120 μmol; this may be effective in:
  a Preventing exchange transfusion in mild cases.
  b Reducing the need for subsequent exchanges in severe ones.

Anaemia. All infants with HDN are prone to anaemia for two reasons:
1 Continuing haemolysis.
2 Depressed erythropoesis for 4−6 weeks after birth.
Serial Hb levels and reticulocyte counts are mandatory to determine the need for top-up tranfusions; Hb should not be allowed to fall below 7−8 g; an absolute reticulocyte count of >200 × 10^9/l indicates good bone marrow function.

Folic acid deficiency. Many infants with HDN become folate deficient due to the increased red cell turnover. Since folate is essential for *all* cell division this may result in impaired growth rather than megaloblastic anaemia. All but the mildest cases should receive folate supplements for the first 3−6 months of life.

Other rhesus haemolytic disease

The other Rh antigens E, e, C, c, can all cause haemolytic disease but rarely produce severe intra-uterine anaemia. Elective delivery near term is indicated, the need for phototherapy and exchange transfusion is dictated by serial bilirubin measurements.

ABO incompatibility (haemolytic disease due to maternal anti-A or anti-B haemolysins of the IgG class)

The condition is different from rhesus incompatibility since the antibodies are naturally occuring and not due to feto-maternal transfusion. It arises when a group O mother carries a group A or (more rarely) a group B fetus, and occurs only in the 10% of such women who have IgG haemolysins. The antigens are weak, the fetus is not severely affected *in utero* and no antenatal investigation or planned delivery are necessary. It may occur in first pregnancies, and subsequent ones are not more severely affected.

Clinical features

ABO incompatability is much more common than rhesus disease. The infant presents with jaundice during the first 2 days (see also Table 22.2). The Coombs' test is negative or only weakly positive. The diagnosis is suspected from the blood groups of mother and baby and is usually confirmed by demonstrating an IgG haemolysin in the mother's serum. Anaemia is not a problem and the prognosis is excellent. The hyperbilirubinaemia is treated as in Rh disease.

Reference

Liley, A.W. (1963) Errors in the assessment of haemolytic disease from amniotic fluid. *American Journal of Obstetrics and Gynecology* **86**, 485–94.

Further reading

Mowat, A.P. (1986) Liver disease in the neonate. In *Textbook of Neonatal Medicine*. N.R.C. Roberton (ed.), Churchill Livingstone, Edinburgh. pp.394–406.
Roberton, N.R.C. (1986) Neonatal Jaundice. In *Recent advances in Paediatrics, No. 8*. S.R. Meadow (ed.), Churchill Livingstone, Edinburgh. pp.157–83.
Whitfield, C.R. (1983) Haemolytic disease of the newborn — a continuing problem. In *Recent Advances in Perinatal Medicine, No. 1*. Chiswick M.L. (ed.), Churchill Livingstone, Edinburgh. pp.95–115.

Chapter 23
Endocrine and Metabolic Disorders in the Newborn

Hypoglycaemia

Hypoglycaemia is usually defined as values <1.5 mmol/l in term babies during the first week and <1.0 mmol/l in premature and SFD babies. Levels <2.0 mmol/l in fullterm infants older than 1 week indicate hypoglycaemia.

Symptoms

1 Those due to the catecholamine response to hypoglycaemia — pallor, sweating and tachycardia, are very rare in neonates.
2 Cardiac effects: bradycardia, hypotension, and heart failure.
3 Apnoea or convulsions — signs of neuroglycopenia — indicate serious hypoglycaemia and require urgent treatment.
Jitteriness is probably not a sign of neuroglycopenia; it is common in SFD infants whether they are hypoglycaemic or not.

Sequelae

A striking feature of neonatal hypoglycaemia is the fact that infants may be asymptomatic with blood glucose values less than 1.0 mmol/l. Only after some hours with such a low blood sugar do apnoea and convulsions occur. This fact has important clinical implications, since it means that routines to detect hypoglycaemia can be designed in the knowledge that transient asymptomatic hypoglycaemia is benign.

Neonates with hypoglycaemic fits or apnoeic attacks may be retarded or have cerebral palsy on follow up.

Causes of hypoglycaemia

There are two main groups of conditions which cause hypoglycaemia in the neonatal period: those due to depleted glycogen stores and those due to hyperinsulinaemia.

269

Depleted glycogen stores

This occurs in small for dates infants. These are dealt with in detail in Chapters 12 and 13.

Prematurity. Very premature infants become hypoglycaemic not only because they are delivered before the glycogen stores are laid down, but if they are ill during the first 1–2 weeks, their calorie intake is often inadequate.

Undernutrition. Even normally-grown infants may become hypoglycaemic on the second to third day of life when they have been difficult to feed and have taken very little milk.

Intrapartum asphyxia. When severe, this will deplete the liver and myocardial glycogen stores in even normal term infants, who will, as a result, become hypoglycaemic during or following resuscitation. In addition to neuroglycopenia, these infants develop heart failure, cardiomegaly, muffled heart sounds, bradycardia and poor peripheral perfusion.

Serious illness of any type. Infants with congenital heart disease or septicaemia may also have blood glucose levels less than 1.0 mmol/l, and develop apnoea or seizures as a result.

Hypoglycaemia due to hyperinsulinaemia

Infants of diabetic mothers (IDM)

If diabetes is inadequately controlled, babies are large for dates with cardiomegaly, splenomegaly, hepatomegaly, a very characteristic plethoric appearance and an increased incidence of malformation. They are at risk from RDS, hypoglycaemia, hypocalcaemia and jaundice. Throughout gestation the babies are exposed to high blood glucose values. They develop hyperinsulinism which persists postnatally. When cut off from the transplacental infusion of glucose, they quickly become hypoglycaemic. Blood glucose levels ≤0.2 mmol/l may be recorded by 90–120 minutes of age. However, the infant has adequate glycogen stores and the defence mechanisms against hypoglycaemia are working. In most IDM the blood glucose rises spontaneously to above 1.0 mmol/l by 4 hours of age. Persisting hypoglycaemia is rare unless the IDM have also suffered from asphyxia or develop RDS. If the blood glucose is still less than 1.0 mmol/l by 4 hours of age, or if symptoms develop, i.v. dextrose is indicated (p.272).

If an IDM is feeding well by 12 hours of age, and has not been hypoglycaemic, he is very unlikely to have any further problems.

Haemolytic disease of the newborn

Neonates with rhesus HDN have islet cell hypertrophy related to the severity of the anaemia at birth. Infants with cord haemoglobin values less than 10 g/l are particularly at risk from hypoglycaemia which commonly occurs as a rebound after exchange transfusion with bank blood, which has a high glucose content.

Unusual causes of neonatal hypoglycaemia

Severe hypoglycaemia with convulsions or apnoea may also occur in:
1 Endocrine deficiences — multiple or single (e.g. growth hormone, ACTH, cortisol, thyroxine).
2 Syndromes with hyperinsulinaemia:
  a Beckwith–Wiedemann syndrome.
  b Islet cell adenoma.
  c Nesidioblastosis.
  d Leucine sensitivity.
  e Infant giant syndrome.
3 Inborn errors of carbohydrate metabolism:
  a Glycogen storage disease.
  b Fructose intolerance: fructose 1:6 diposphatase deficiency.
  c Galactosaemia.
4 Aminoacidopathies:
  a Maple syrup urine disease.
  b Propionic acidaemia.
  c Methylmalonic acidaemia.
  d Tyrosinosis.
These should only be considered if there is some other diagnostic lead, or if hypoglycaemia is persistent.

Management of hypoglycaemia

The details of the detection, prevention and treatment of hypoglycaemia in SFD and premature babies are given in Chapters 12 and 13.

Prevention

Infants at risk should have their blood glucose monitored by Dextrostix at the stated times (Chapter 13). Appropriate feeds should be given to infants likely to tolerate enteral nutrition (pp.106–7); otherwise infuse 10% dextrose intravenously.

Treatment of asymptomatic hypoglycaemia

Send off a blood sample to the laboratory to confirm the diagnosis if detection was based on Dextrostix. Immediately give the next milk feed due by tube if necessary and check the Dextrostix 1 hour later; if the Dextrostix is now >1.5 mmol/l continue feeding as before. If the Dextrostix is still ≤1.4 mmol/l, give a single dose of 0.5 g/kg of 10% dextrose i.v. immediately, followed by an infusion of 10% dextrose at 60 ml/kg/24 hours.

Treatment of symptomatic hypoglycaemia

Confirm the diagnosis and give 1 g/kg of 10% dextrose i.v. at once followed by i.v. infusion as above. Aim to keep the glucose >1.5 mmol/l; occasionally it is necessary to give 15–20% dextrose to maintain this. Drugs such as hydrocortisone or diazoxide are rarely indicated.

Always maintain enteral feeding if possible in hypoglycaemic infants. Once the blood glucose is stable, the i.v. can be discontinued gradually, and the oral intake built up to maintenance (pp.106–7).

Neonatal hyperglycaemia

Neonatal diabetes mellitus

The neonate, usually SFD, loses weight and has polyuria. Hyperglycaemia, acidaemia and dehydration occur but ketosis is rare. The infants are exquisitely sensitive to exogenous insulin, 0.5–1.0 unit of insulin twice a day is often all that is required to control the disease. Within 1–2 months the infant recovers completely, and insulin can be discontinued.

Iatrogenic

If premature infants receive 10% dextrose infused at rates which give them more than 6 mg/kg/minute, it may exceed their capacity to metabolize it. They then develop glycosuria with an osmotic diuresis and dehydration. The hyperglycaemia predisposes them to bacterial and fungal sepsis. In these babies the concentration of the glucose infusion should be reduced.

The neonate with ambiguous genitalia

Causes

Female pseudohermaphroditism (i.e. a genetic female who is masculinized):
• Maternal androgen/progesterone therapy
• Congenital adrenal hyperplasia (CAH) (see below)
Male pseudohermaphroditism (i.e. a genetic male who is feminized):
• Extreme perineo-scrotal hypospadias
• Testosterone biosynthetic defects
• Partial testicular feminization syndrome
• Rare variants of CAH
Other genetic defects:
• Sex chromosome mosaics
• True hermaphrodites

Assessment

Only male babies have testes; therefore whether or not these are present is a key factor in deciding which urgent investigation to proceed with.

Other factors to assess immediately are:
1 Whether or not the infant has CAH (see below). What is the genetic sex of the infant? Do the karyotype, since buccal smears are inaccurate in the neonate.
2 In genetic males, can the external genitalia ever be fashioned into a sexually functional penis? If not, rear the child as a female.

Once these factors have been established, and the delicate discussions with the parents have been undertaken, the more complex investigations which may be required can then be carried out.

Congenital adrenal hyperplasia (incidence 1:5000)

Two main enzyme defects: absent 21α-hydroxylase (>90%), absent 11β-hydroxylase ($\simeq$10%).

21α-hydroxylase deficency usually presents with virilization and/or a salt-losing state; 11 β-hydroxylase deficiency with virilization and/or hypertension.

The diagnosis is confirmed by demonstrating a raised plasma level of 17α-hydroxyprogesterone (in 21α-hydroxylase deficiency) or 11β-deoxycortisol (in 11 β-hydroxylase deficiency).

While waiting for the results of these assays, virilized females should have daily plasma and urinary electrolyte measurements to check for salt loss.

Male neonates will present with vomiting, weight loss and Addisonian crisis unless someone has astutely noted minor increases in scrotal and nipple pigmentation or in penile growth. Cases of either sex who develop symptoms need i.v. normal saline and glucose plus 25–50 mg of i.v. hydrocortisone as a matter of urgency. Once the diagnosis is established, maintenance treatment is with 2.5 mg bd of hydrocortisone: add 0.05–0.1 mg of 9α fluorocortisol daily plus 2–4 g NaCl daily in salt losers.

Neonatal thyroid disease

Congenital hypothyroidism (incidence 1:3500)

(Neonatal screening routine p.87).
Most hypothyroid neonates have small or absent thyroid glands. However, if a neonate has a goitre, maternal ingestion of goitrogens (iodides, antithyroid drugs) should be sought, but full investigation of goitres due to inherited defects can be carried out when the child is older. If hypothyroidism is detected, irrespective of the aetiology, give 10 μg/kg of l-thyroxine daily, but check the diagnosis at 1 year.

Neonatal thyrotoxicosis

This is due to transplacental passage of thyroid-stimulating immunoglobulins, and only develops in the infants of the small percentage of mothers who have high titres. The neonate is usually <2.5 kg at birth, and may develop signs of thyrotoxicosis including:
• Tachycardia, progressing to heart failure
• Exophthalmos and lid lag
• Extreme jitteriness
• Vomiting, diarrhoea, poor weight gain
• Sweating
• Goitre (with a bruit) which may obstruct the trachea

The disease is life-threatening. Initial treatment should be propranolol, Lugol's iodine, and propylthiouracil. Digitalization should also be considered. As the level of thyroid-stimulating immunoglobulins declines, antithyroid drugs can be discontinued usually by 2−3 months of age. The infants often have mild neurological abnormalities on follow-up.

Inborn errors of metabolism

Galactosaemia (incidence 1:40 000−60 000)

Usually deficiency of galactose−1−phosphate uridyl transferase. Autosomal recessive; antenatal detection possible; neonatal screening possible.

Affected infants, who must be receiving milk to develop symptoms, present with:

- Vomiting, occasionally diarrhoea
- Lethargy and hypotonia
- Poor weight gain
- Persistent jaundice
- Hepatosplenomegaly
- Cataracts (occasionally)

Many cases, however, become seriously ill and die from septicaemia before galactosaemia is diagnosed. Galactosaemia is very likely if an infant with these symptoms has a reducing substance (Clinitest +ve, Clinistix -ve) in his urine.

Start any infant suspected of galactosaemia on a lactose-free milk (Galactomin, or Pregestimil) as soon as possible while confirming the diagnosis by assaying galactose−1−phosphate-uridyl-transferase in his red cells.

Amino-acid disorders

The majority of these do not cause symptoms in the neonatal period but if they do with neurological symptoms, or because of the family history, the appropriate formula should be started (Table 23.1).

Phenylketonuria (incidence approx. 1:10 000)

Deficiency of phenylalanine hydroxylase; autosomal recessive; antenatal detection not possible; neonatal screening routine. For details of neonatal management see Chapter 10.

Table 23.1. Formulae for amino-acid disorders.

Disorder	Milk
Phenylketonuria	Albumaid, Lofenelac, Minafen
Maple syrup urine disease	MSUD Aid
Homocystinuria	Albumaid — methionine low

Organic acidaemias (propionic acidaemia, methylmalonic acidaemia), Non-ketotic hyperglycinaemia, Maple syrup urine disease

These are a group of autosomal recessive disorders each with an incidence of about 1:250 000; some can be detected antenatally. In their acute neonatal forms they have a comparatively uniform clinical picture with:

1 Consanguineous parents with previous unexplained neonatal deaths.
2 Profound CNS disturbance within 48–72 hours of delivery, usually, but not always after starting milk feeds, with lethargy, poor feeding, alterations of tone and fits.
3 Apnoea.
4 Profound metabolic acidaemia (base deficit > 15 mmol/l) and ketosis.
5 Hypoglycaemia.
6 Thrombocytopenia and neutropenia.
7 Varying patterns of amino-acidaemia and amino-aciduria.
8 Coma, usually progressing to death.

Initial resuscitation and urgent diagnosis is important because:
1 Some of the conditions are treatable by appropriate dietary restriction or large doses of vitamin coenzymes (Table 23.2).
2 Many of the conditions are detectable by antenatal amniocentesis in the next pregnancy.

The chemical expertise required for the diagnosis of these disorders is confined to specialized laboratories, and appropriate plasma

Table 23.2. Organic acidaemias.

Disorder	Treatment available	Likely outcome
Maple syrup urine disease	Special formula	Good with early treatment
Isovaleric acidaemia	Low protein diet	Fair
Propionic acidaemia	Low protein diet	Poor
Methylmalonic acidaemia	Low protein diet, B_{12} in large doses	Poor unless B_{12} responsive
Non-ketotic hyperglycinaemia	Nil	Hopeless

and urine samples should be sent to them as soon as possible after the clinical problem is recognized.

While establishing whether long-term therapy is feasible, initially treat the baby with IPPV; correct his acidosis, stop the protein intake and consider removing abnormal metabolites by exchange transfusion or peritoneal dialysis.

Urea cycle disorders (hyperammonaemias) (incidence approx. 1:250 000)

Deficiences of all the urea cycle enzmes are described: autosomal recessive or sex-linked recessive; antenatal detection is possible (Table 23.3).

These present like the organic acidaemias; however, acidaemia and ketosis are absent and there is gross hyperammonaemia (>1000 μg/100 ml [590 μmol/l]).

Table 23.3. Hyperammonaemias.

Disorder	Genetics	Outcome
Ornithine transcarbamylase deficiency	Sex-linked	Fatal in males Fair in females
Argininosuccinic aciduria	Recessive	Fair
Citrullinaemia	Recessive	Poor with neonatal forms
Carbamyl phosphate synthetase deficiency	Recessive	Poor
Hyperargininaemia	Recessive	Poor

Treatment

Treatment involves reducing or stopping the protein intake, lowering the blood ammonia levels by exchange transfusion or dialysis, and preventing ammonia release by gut bacteria with oral neomycin and laxatives.

In infants with the acute neonatal forms of these diseases, the long-term management is stormy and rarely successful.

Further reading

Barnes, N.D. (1986) Endocrine Disorders. In *Textbook of Neonatology*, N.R.C. Roberton (ed.), Churchill Livingstone, Edinburgh. pp.623−43.

Stanbury, J.B., Wyngaarden, J.B., Fredrickson, D.S., Goldstein, J.S. & Brown, M.S. (1983) *The Metabolic Basis of Inherited Disease*, 5th edn. McGraw Hill, New York.

Chapter 24
Genito-Urinary Disease in the Newborn

Renal Disease

Failure to pass urine after birth

In an apparently well infant the causes and treatment are indicated in Table 24.1. In an ill infant anuria will probably be due to pre-renal or intrinsic renal failure.

Table 24.1. Failure to pass urine after birth.

Cause	Clinical features	Action
Passed unobserved in labour ward	Well baby, normal examination	Wait and see
Lethal renal malformation	Oligohydramnios, 'Potter's' facies, usually severe respiratory distress (pulmonary hypoplasia), no bladder palpable	Ultrasound, pass catheter
Obstructive uropathy	Large bladder and/or kidneys	Pass catheter, ultrasound, micturating cystogram

Haematuria

This is uncommon in neonates; the commonest cause of pink staining on the nappy is the presence of urates. The colour disappears on acidification and heating. In the female, the blood may be vaginal in origin (withdrawal of maternal oestrogens). Haematuria, confirmed by microscopy can be caused by:
1 Coagulopathy:
 a DIC (p.291).
 b Haemorrhagic disease (p.290).
2 Vascular:
 a Renal vein thrombosis (see below).
 b Renal artery thrombosis or embolus.
3 Acute tubular necrosis secondary to circulatory insufficiency (p.280).

4 Traumatic, e.g. following suprapubic aspiration.
5 Urinary tract infection (p.181).
6 Obstructive uropathy (p.284).
7 Congenital cystic disorders and hydronephrosis (p.284).
8 Tumours (very rare).
 a Mesoblastic nephroma.
 b Wilms' tumour.
 c Angioma.

Proteinuria

Low-grade proteinuria is normally present in the first week of life. Other causes:
- Conditions listed for haematuria
- Birth asphyxia
- Congenital nephrotic syndrome (very rare)
- Congenital and neonatal infections
- Drugs, e.g. mercury compounds (very rare)

Urinary tract infection (p.181)

Renal vein thrombosis

This is due to stasis associated with hypovolaemic states and/or polycythaemia. The most likely predisposing conditions are:
- Asphyxia/hypoxia/hypotension
- Dehydration
- DIC
- Maternal diabetes (polycythaemia)

Clinically, the infant presents with enlarged, smooth kidneys, haematuria, and oliguria or anuria. Treatment is that of the underlying disorder and expectant management of the renal failure.

Renal failure

Failure of renal function is suggested by the following clinical and biochemical findings:
- Urine output <25 ml/kg/day, i.e. <1 ml/kg/hour
- Serum potassium >7 mmol/l and rising
- Blood urea >10 mmol/l and rising by >1 mmol/l/day
- Creatinine rising by >50 μmol/l/day

Aetiology (Table 24.2)

The commonest cause of reduced urine output is underperfusion of normal kidneys, i.e. pre-renal uraemia. This can result from hypovolaemia and/or hypotension. If the ischaemia is severe or prolonged it leads to acute tubular necrosis (ATN) with acute renal failure.

Investigation

If there is oliguria, pre-renal failure can be differentiated from renal failure since functioning kidneys can concentrate urine, retain sodium and excrete metabolites (Table 24.3).

The presence of renal mass(es) indicates hydronephrosis, cystic

Table 24.2. Causes of renal failure in the neonate.

Pre-renal

  Birth asphyxia
  Postnatal hypoxia
  Hypovolaemia secondary to:
    Blood loss (before or after birth)
    Fluid loss (through skin, gastro-intestinal tract or kidney)
    Hypoalbuminaemia
    Inadequate fluid intake

  Hypotension secondary to:
    Septic shock
    Drugs (e.g. tolazoline)
    Cardiac failure
    Hypoxia, acidaemia

Renal

  Congenital renal malformations

    Renal agenesis/hypoplasia
    Renal dysplasia
    Infantile polycystic disease
    Acute tubular or cortical necrosis secondary to pre-renal failure

  Vascular
    Renal vein thrombosis
    Renal artery thrombosis or embolus
    Disseminated intra-vascular coagulation

Post-renal

  Obstructive uropathy (see Table 24.5)

Table 24.3. Laboratory aids in the differential diagnosis of pre-renal failure and acute tubular necrosis.

	Pre-renal failure	Acute tubular necrosis
Urinary sodium (mmol/l)	<10	>40
Urine/plasma osmolality	>2	<1.1
Urine/plasma urea	>20	<5
Urine/plasma creatinine	>40	<5

disorder or renal vein thrombosis; these can be differentiated by ultrasound. An enlarged bladder suggests obstructive uropathy.

Management of pre-renal failure

Early treatment of pre-renal failure includes:
1 Blood volume correction with blood, plasma, or electrolyte solutions in aliquots of 10−20 ml/kg.
2 Dopamine infusion (5−20µg/kg/minute) for persisting hypotension; it also improves renal blood flow.
3 If oliguria persists after correcting blood volume and pressure, give frusemide 1−5 mg/kg intravenously.
Lack of diuretic response after these measures is highly suggestive of intrinsic renal failure.

Management of established renal failure

Meticulous attention to control of fluid and electrolyte balance, regular weighing once or twice a day, twice daily serum electrolytes, and accurate measurement of urinary output and composition are essential.

Fluids. Restrict to insensible water losses + urinary output, if any. Insensible loss varies from 20−30 ml/kg/day in the fullterm infant to 60−100 ml/kg/day in the preterm infant under a radiant heater or phototherapy.

Sodium. Restrict sodium intake to 0.3 mmol/kg/24 hours or less provided plasma level is >120 mmol/l. If plasma sodium falls below 120 mmol/l correct it to 125 over 1−2 hours ([125−plasma Na] × 0.7 × body-weight in kg).

Acidosis. Correct metabolic acidosis with THAM or bicarbonate to maintain H^+ concentration <60 nmol/l (pH >7.25).

Potassium. Stop potassium intake. Levels >7 mmol/l without marked ECG changes should be treated with rectal Resonium $1-4$ times daily. Use Resonium A (sodium salt) if plasma sodium normal; if hypernatraemic use the calcium salt. Hyperkalaemia with major ECG changes needs urgent treatment with intravenous calcium gluconate 100 mg/kg (1 ml 10% solution) and bicarbonate 2 mmol/kg; or i.v. glucose and insulin (3 g glucose/1u insulin). Consider peritoneal dialysis.

Antibiotics. Infection is common: blood levels of nephrotoxic or ototoxic antibiotics must be measured.

Anaemia. Give transfusions as packed red cells to avoid the infusion of plasma with a high potassium concentration.

Dialysis. Peritoneal dialysis in the neonate is relatively straightforward but should only be undertaken in experienced centres. The indications are:
1 Fluid overload not responding to fluid restriction.
2 Hyperkalaemia with ECG changes or rapidly rising levels.
3 Severe and uncontrollable metabolic acidosis (base deficit >15 mmol/l).

Congenital malformations

Congenital renal malformations are summarized in Table 24.4.

Obstructive uropathy

Obstruction to flow may occur anywhere in the urinary tract; the effects depend upon the degree and site of the obstruction (Table 24.5). Any obstructive lesion may lead to urinary tract infection.

Genitalia

Inguinal hernia and hydrocele

Indirect inguinal herniae and hydroceles are common, especially in preterm infants.

Table 24.4. Features of some congenital renal malformations.

Condition	Incidence	M:F Ratio	Clinical features	Inheritance
Bilateral renal agenesis	1/4000	2/1	Oligohydramnios, Potter's facies, pulmonary hypoplasia: lethal	Usually sporadic but can be AR, AD, or sex-linked
Unilateral renal agenesis	1/2500	?	Usually asymptomatic; increased incidence of other renal and extra-renal malformations	Dominant form may be expressed uni- or bilaterally in the same family
Renal hypoplasia	?	3/1	renal failure in childhood	Rarely familial
Cystic/ dysplastic kidneys	?	2/1	bilateral = lethal unilateral = multicystic kidney; 90% have other urinary tract anomalies	Usually sporadic
Polycystic disease (adult form)	1/500	1/1	Usually asymptomatic in neonate. May have enlarged cystic kidneys. +ve family history	AD
Polcystic disease (neonatal form)*	1/6000	0.5/1	Respiratory problems at birth. Huge cystic kidneys. Renal failure	AR

AR = Autosomal recessive   AD = Autosomal dominant
*NB. Infantile form may present later as renal failure and/or flank masses.

Isolated hydrocele

Presents as a soft, non-tender, translucent swelling in the scrotum which may wax and wane with crying (communicating hydrocele), but sometimes becomes huge. Hydroceles disappear without treatment.

Hernia with or without hydrocele

Presents as a lump in the groin or scrotum which may appear on crying and disappear when the infant is relaxed; it can usually be reduced. The internal ring is narrow and there is always a risk of incarceration. Treatment is by elective surgery when the infant is fit. If incarcerated, reduction can usually be achieved under sedation.

Table 24.5. Obstructive uropathy in the neonate.

Site	Lesion	Features	Outcome
Urethral meatus	Stenosis	May be associated with hypospadias (p.285)	Good
Urethra	Atresia	Rare, may be associated with agenetic or dysplastic kidneys. Otherwise gross dilatation of whole urinary tract	Fatal
	Posterior urethral valves	Commonest lower urinary tract obstruction. Large bladder, hydroureters and hydronephroses. May have poor urinary stream but good stream does not exclude diagnosis	Requires early correction. Outlook fair
Bladder	'Prune belly' syndrome	Abdominal wall wrinkled like a prune due to absent abdominal muscles. Large bladder and ureters, hydronephrosis. Almost always male, cryptorchid	Fair outlook. Renal failure in some
Ureter	Atresia or stricture	Usually seen with unilateral multicystic kidney	Good if other kidney normal
Pelviureteric junction		The commonest uropathy, hydronephrosis, bilateral in 20%	Good if renal function is reasonable

Undescended testicles

One or both testes are undescended in about 30% of LBW infants but only in 3–4% of fullterm ones.

Unilateral

Not uncommon, but remember that this may be a retractile testis. No immediate action is necessary but if it has not descended by 1 year it will not do so. Orchidopexy is then indicated before 5 years.

Bilateral

In this case ask the following questions:
1 Could this be some form of intersex, i.e. is there severe hypospadias, hypoplastic scrotum? (See p.273).
2 Is the baby otherwise normal? Could this be a dysmorphic syndrome?

Torsion

Testicular torsion is usually extra-vaginal with the entire tunica vaginalis and its contents torted causing infarction; it may happen antenatally. It presents as a hard, discoloured, non-tender mass which does not transilluminate. Urgent surgery is recommended, although rarely successful in saving the testicle.

Hypospadias

Overall incidence 3.2:1000, and the recurrence risk is about 11%, being most likely with the more severe forms. There are three components:
1 Abnormally placed meatus:
  a Glandular ⎫ mild forms, the most common and occurring as an
  b Coronal   ⎬ isolated abnormality.
  c Mid-shaft ⎭
  d Peno-scrotal ⎫ severe forms, see ambiguous genitalia (p.273).
  e Perineal   ⎭
2 Incomplete development of the prepuce, common to all forms.
3 Chordee (ventral bending of the penis), best described as mild, moderate or severe, present in about one third of the milder forms and all the severe ones.

Management

No immediate treatment is needed. Inspect the meatus for stenosis and observe the urinary stream. Do not circumcise. Corrective surgery should be done before the boy goes to school.

Chapter 25
Neonatal Haematology

Anaemia in the neonate

Acute neonatal anaemia

Pallor in the first few hours of life is due to severe asphyxia or anaemia (or both); all pale infants must have their haemoglobin estimated, and if anaemia is present it may be due to:

1 HDN, e.g. rhesus (p.264).
2 Haemorrhage:
  a From damaged placental vessels.
  b From abruptio or placenta paevia.
  c Feto-maternal haemorrhage.
  d Twin to twin transfusion.
  e Fetal or neonatal haemorrhage (ruptured liver, giant cephalhaematoma).
  f Rarities, e.g. α thalassaemia, congenital hypoplastic anaemia.

ASSESSMENT OF EARLY ANAEMIA

History

Was there excessive vaginal blood loss during labour?

Examination

1 Check the placenta for the presence of abnormal vessels.
2 Is there a twin-twin transfusion.
3 Are there any signs of a neonatal haemorrhage?
4 Check the baby's pulse and respiration — tachycardia, and tachypnoea are signs of a massive haemorrhage.
5 Blood pressure — always!
6 Is there hepatosplenomegaly (extra-medullary haemopoiesis) suggesting a more chronic cause of the anaemia?

INVESTIGATION

Immediate

1 Haemoglobin or PCV measurement: remember these take time to fall after acute haemorrhage.
2 pH and blood gases: these are good emergency tests for the hypoxaemia and acidaemia which follow tissue hypoperfusion.
3 Group and cross match 1 unit of fresh blood.

Later

1 Full blood count, platelet count, Coombs' test.
2 Kleihauer test (for fetal RBC) on mother.
3 Serology for congenital infection: haemoglobin electrophoresis
4 Bone marrow.

TREATMENT

Acute blood loss

Insert an umbilical arterial catheter for easy monitoring and sampling. Give oxygen if necessary, and correct acid base abnormalities. Transfuse the baby immediately — in the labour ward if necessary. If he is in poor condition give 15–20 ml/kg of uncross-matched 0 negative blood over 5–10 minutes. If the infant remains pale, hypotensive and acidotic repeat the transfusion over 15–20 minutes. Aim to achieve a normal blood pressure, pH and a haemoglobin $\geq$ 12 g/100 ml. Up to 50 ml/kg may need to be transfused to achieve this.

Chronic blood loss

If a very anaemic neonate (Hb$\leq$8g) is asymptomatic, or is in heart failure, or has developed hydrops (p.319) this suggests that he has suffered some form of chronic haemorrhage, and has reacted to it.

In all these situations a single volume (80 ml/kg) exchange transfusion using packed cells is the safest way of raising the haemoglobin without exacerbating the heart failure. With milder anaemia (8–12 g/100 ml) a top up transfusion of 20–30 ml/kg can be given under diuretic cover.

Chronic neonatal anaemia

The conditions listed in Table 25.1 may cause the haemoglobin to fall below 10 g/l in an otherwise well neonate. The conditions usually present with some more typical feature but occasionally they just present with anaemia.

In an anaemic baby, after excluding conditions 1, 4, 5 and 7, it is reasonable to assume that he either lacked his placental transfusion, or had an unrecognized perinatal bleed. If the haemoglobin is less than 10 g/l he needs a transfusion of 20−30 ml/kg under diuretic cover, but if his haemoglobin is above 10 g/l, give iron supplements. The haemoglobin should rise but if it does not, or continues to fall, investigation for the rare conditions (6 and 8) should be carried out.

Anaemia of prematurity

The haemoglobin falls to 8−9 g/l by 6−8 weeks of age in many infants who weigh less than 1.5 kg at birth. The cause is not known, but it is probably multifactorial. Folic acid, vitamin E, and iron deficiency plus iatrogenic blood loss have all been suggested, but are unproven, and the most important factor may just be that, in the absence of

Table 25.1.   Chronic neonatal anaemia.

Cause	Diagnosis
1 Mild rhesus or ABO haemolytic disease of the newborn — insufficient to cause jaundice	Maternal history, Coombs' test; antibody studies on the mother
2 Perinatal fetal haemorrhage — not presenting acutely	See pp.286−8
3 Small or absent placental transfusion at delivery	Impossible to diagnose retrospectively
4 Chronic ongoing blood loss especially from GI tract (rare)	Clinical examination, stool and urine analysis
5 Chronic infection, especially UTI and occasionally congenital infections	Clinical examination, urine analysis and WBC; cultures
6 Rare red cell abnormalities: Spherocytosis Enzyme deficiences (e.g. G-6-PD) Haemoglobinopathies	 Blood film, family studies. Enzyme assay, raised reticulocyte count Haemoglobin electrophoresis, raised reticulocyte count, family studies
7 Drug-induced	Maternal history.
8 Congenital marrow aplasias or leukaemia	Clinical abnormalities, bone marrow. Extremely rare

erythropoietin, the premature baby's growth may outstrip his marrow's capacity to produce enough red cells to fill the vascular tree: anaemia results.

Management

Check the haemoglobin and reticulocyte count weekly on all VLBW survivors and supplement them with iron (50 mg $FeSO_4$ daily) vitamin E (10 mg daily) and folic acid (0.2 mg daily); if more than $150-200\times10^9/l$ reticulocytes appear the haemoglobin will rise spontaneously.

However, a small number of babies whose haemoglobin falls below 7–8 g/l will develop lethargy, poor feeding, mild tachycardia and tachypnoea. A 20 ml/kg transfusion of packed cells can then be given.

Neonatal polycythaemia

Newborn infants become polycythaemic in the following situations:
• Recipients of twin-to-twin transfusion
• Recipients of a large placental transfusion
• Fetal growth retardation
• Infants of diabetic mothers
• Rarities, e.g. neonatal thyrotoxicosis, Beckwith's syndrome

Diagnosis

Polycythaemia should only be diagnosed if the venous PCV is >65–70%; capillary PCVs may be 15% higher than the true central PCV. As the true PCV rises above 65% the viscosity of blood increases markedly, and the following problems have been attributed to this:
• CNS depression, fits and cortical venous thrombosis
• Heart failure
• Respiratory distress and cyanosis
• Jaundice
• Hypoglycaemia
• Hypocalcaemia
• Renal vein thrombosis

Treatment

Some authorities recommend therapy for all infants with a venous PCV > 65–70%. However, therapy is probably only needed if the first three symptoms listed above develop, or if the venous PCV exceeds 80%. The PCV is lowered by carrying out a 20–30 ml/kg exchange transfusion with plasma.

Haemorrhagic disorders

The neonate, particularly if born prematurely, is deficient in all the factors involved in the intrinsic clotting mechanism with the exception of factors V and VIII. The levels rise to adult values within a few weeks.

Coagulation of the neonate is assessed with the following tests:
1 Activated partial thromboplastin time (Fig. 25.1).
2 Prothrombin time (Fig. 25.1).
3 Thrombin time — assesses fibrinogen and antithrombins including heparin and fibrin degradation products.

Haemorrhagic disease of the newborn

This is due to a deficiency of factors II, VII, IX and X. It presents on

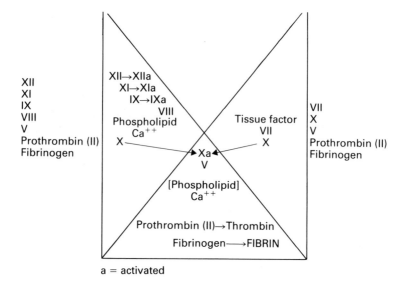

a = activated

Fig. 25.1. Activated partial thromboplastin time (APTT) and prothrombin time (PT). Those portions of the coagulation mechanism measured by the APTT are in the triangle on the left; those measured by PT, in the triangle on the right. Listed on the left are the factors that influence the APTT and on the right, those that influence the PT. (From Abildgaard, 1981.)

the second—fourth day of life with haemorrhage from the cord stump, haematemesis and melaena, ecchymoses, epistaxes or scalp haemorrhage. The infant may also bleed from puncture sites or a circumcision. The prothrombin time and the activated partial thromboplastin time (APTT) are very prolonged, but the thrombin time and fibrinogen level are usually normal.

If this disease develops, give 1–5 mg of i.v. vitamin K stat. An immediate blood transfusion is usually indicated if the infant is shocked; more gradual correction of anaemia by exchange transfusion should be used if the infant is anaemic, but has had time to haemodilute.

The condition can and should be prevented by routinely giving all babies 1 mg of vitamin K at birth.

Disseminated intravascular coagulation

This may develop in neonates with severe birth asphyxia, septicaemia, hypothermia, hypotension, hypoxaemia or acidaemia. It usually presents as petechial bleeding into the skin, or oozing from puncture sites, but haemorrhage may occur anywhere.

The intravascular coagulation consumes platelets, factors II, V, VIII, XIII and fibrinogen, leaving the infant with a bleeding diathesis.

Diagnosis

The PT, APTT and thrombin time are all prolonged, and there is an increased titre of fibrin degradation products. The platelet count may fall below $100 \times 10^9/l$ ($100\,000/mm^3$), and damaged RBC are seen on examination of a blood film.

Treatment

Treat the underlying disease. Replace deficient clotting factors by transfusion of fresh frozen plasma (10–15 ml/kg), or platelets. In severely affected infants consider exchange transfusion with fresh blood.

Congenital deficiences of coagulation factors

These may all present in the neonatal period, usually with haemorrhage following surgical procedures such as circumcision. Haemophilia (factor VIII deficiency) is present in 90% of such cases.

Neonatal thrombocytopenia

This usually presents with purpura, ecchymoses or a large cephalhaematoma. Bleeding from other sites is comparatively rare. Thrombocytopenia is found in the following conditions in the neonatal period:

- DIC (p.291)
- Sepsis (p.177)
- Haemangiomatosis
- Congenital infection
- Maternal idiopathic thrombocytopenia or DLE with transplacental passage of anti-platelet IgG
- Iso-immune thrombocytopenia — the mother making antibodies to antigenically different fetal platelets
- In association with Rh HDN:
- Marrow abnormalities (leukaemia, hypoplasia)
- Drugs (administered to mother or infants — quinidine, thiazides)
- Inherited abnormalities, e.g. Wiskott–Aldrich
- Methylmalonic acidaemia, etc. (p.276)

The differential diagnosis can usually be established easily from the history, clinical examination, coagulation studies and bone marrow cytology.

Treatment

Although most studies of neonatal thrombocytopenia report a high morbidity from intracranial haemorrhage, this probably occurs intrapartum, so that if thrombocytopenia is anticipated, the baby should be delivered by caesarean section. Neonatal thrombocytopenia with no signs other than some purpura or a few petechiae does not need treatment. If major bleeding occurs, platelet transfusion should be considered. If the thrombocytopenia is due to platelet antibodies an exchange transfusion may be more appropriate.

Reference

Abildgaard, C.F. (1981) Diseases of coagulation. In *Haematology of Infancy and Child-hood*, 2nd edn., D.G. Nathan & F.A. Oski (eds.), W.B. Saunders & Co., Philadelphia.

Further reading

Oski, F.A., Naiman, J.L. (1982) *Haematologic Problems in the Newborn*. W.B. Saunders & Co., Philadelphia.

Chapter 26
Orthopaedic Problems and Structural Malformations

Hare lip and cleft palate

Incidence: hare lip with or without cleft palate 1:600, more common in males; cleft palate alone 1:2500, more common in females.

Aetiology

1 There is a hereditary tendency with the following recurrence risks:
- Father affected, 3%
- Mother affected, 14%
- One affected sibling, 4%
- Two affected siblings, 10%

2 Drugs, e.g. phenytoin have been implicated.

3 The defects can be associated with chromosomal and other dysmorphic syndromes. Always check for other malformations in affected babies.

Clinical features

Hare lip varies from a barely perceptible groove to a complete cleft extending to the floor of the nose. Single clefts are about twice as common as bilateral ones, the latter nearly always pass through the alveolar ridge and are associated with a cleft palate. Mid-line lip clefts are very rare.

Cleft palate varies from a bifid uvula and a mid-line cleft in the soft palate to one extending over the whole length of both hard and soft palates, the defect in the hard palate can be uni- or bilateral if associated with hare lip.

Management

The parents should be seen urgently. It is very useful to have a set of photographs of a baby before and after surgery to demonstrate the excellent cosmetic results.

Feeding

Hare lip or cleft soft palate alone rarely cause problems, but in severe
defects sucking and swallowing may be difficult. With a large palatal
defect a prosthetic plate promotes maxillary growth and facilitates
feeding. Try using a large hole teat or one with a flange; occasionally
the infant has to be spoon-fed. Breast-feeding is perfectly possible.

Later management

1 Lip repair is done at 3−6 months but palatal closure is usually
delayed until about 9 months.
2 Speech therapy may be required for children with cleft palate.
3 Infants with cleft palate are prone to otitis media.

Congenital dislocation of the hip (CDH)

Aetiology

Factors to consider are:
1 Genetic — a positive family history.
2 Sex — females are about four times more commonly affected than
males.
3 Intra-uterine malposition, e.g. breech presentation increases the
risk fourteenfold; CDH is more common with oligohydramnios and is
associated with talipes.
5 CDH is common when there is neuro-muscular imbalance, e.g.
myelomeningocele.

Incidence

This is hard to determine. In an unscreened population the incidence
of dislocated hips at 1 year is about 0.1% whereas the incidence of
unstable and dislocated hips discovered on routine neonatal screening
is about 1% of which 50−75% are dislocatable and will probably
resolve with or without treatment. Despite routine neonatal hip
examination:
1 Some dislocated hips are missed.
2 The incidence of late diagnosis has not fallen to the extent that
would be expected if most cases were detectable in the neonatal
period.

Diagnosis

The examination is described in detail in Chapter 7.

Management

This remains controversial since most unstable (dislocatable) hips resolve spontaneously. Some advocate immediate splintage of all unstable hips, whereas others favour a period of observation, only splinting those that remain abnormal. General agreement exists on the following principles of management:

1 Do not regard neonatal screening as a once and for all test. The hips should be evaluated as part of all routine infant examinations.

2 Dislocat*able* hips, if not splinted immediately, must be carefully rechecked; if they remain unstable after 3−6 weeks they should be splinted.

3 Dislocat*ed* hips should always be splinted in abduction for 6−12 weeks after birth with careful orthopaedic follow-up.

4 Beware of hips with limited abduction since these may be dislocated. They should be followed until movements are full or a definite diagnosis is made.

5 Irreducible dislocations nearly always need surgical reduction.

6 'Clicking' hips are normal.

Abnormalities of the feet

Neonates often have minor foot abnormalities due to intra-uterine compression. Provided the feet and ankles can be put through a normal range of movements there is no need for concern and the malpositions will rapidly correct themselves spontaneously. Severe deformities, however, need early treatment if normal walking is to be achieved.

Metatarsus varus (metatarsus adductus, hooked forefoot)

Metatarsus varus is when the forefoot is turned medially; most cases are 'positional'; the forefoot can be abducted beyond the neutral point and requires no treatment.

Talipes (clubfoot)

Talipes calcaneo-valgus is common and is due to the foot being compressed by the uterus onto the anterior surface of the tibia. The foot can almost always be corrected beyond the normal position and no treatment is needed.

Talipes equino-varus (TEV)

Incidence 1.2:1000 rising twentyfold if a first degree relative is affected. Males are three times more commonly affected than females; 50% are bilateral. True TEV is serious and requires early treatment. There are three structural elements to TEV:
1 Equinus position of the ankle.
2 Varus (inversion) of the hindfoot.
3 Varus (adduction) of the forefoot.
The diagnosis is made when the deformity cannot be over-corrected, i.e. the foot cannot become plantigrade.

Management

As soon as possible after birth strap the foot in the best position. This will correct many cases but long-term plaster casts and splints followed by corrective surgery may be needed.

Fractures

Bones can be broken during delivery, although the incidence of fractures has fallen with improved obstetric management. The bones most liable to injury are the clavicle, humerus and femur. The infants most at risk are:
1 Breech presentations, particularly with extended legs.
2 Very large infants, particularly if there is cephalo-pelvic disproportion or shoulder dystocia.
3 Difficult forceps deliveries.

Clinical features

Sometimes a snap is heard or felt at delivery. After birth there is swelling and sometimes bruising over the affected bone; crepitus may be felt. Movements of the affected limb are obviously painful. Diagnosis is confirmed by X-ray.

Fractured clavicle is commonest in breech delivery or with shoulder dystocia. Erb's palsy (p.223) commonly coexists.

Fractured humerus is usually in the mid-shaft particularly in breech delivery with extended arms.

Fractured femur is commonest in breech deliveries and is also in mid-shaft.

Skull. See p.221.

Treatment

Although various immobilization procedures have been advocated, most fractures heal very well without interference and there is an amazing capacity for spontaneous re-alignment. Take care in moving the affected part and provide analgesia if the baby is in obvious pain. The prognosis for fractures is excellent.

Occasionally, pathological fractures which may be prenatal, are seen in association with osteogenesis imperfecta; X-rays show abundant callus formation. The severe neonatal form presents as a dwarf with multiple fractures (p.300).

Rickets (osteopenia of prematurity)

During the last trimester of pregnancy large amounts of calcium and phosphorus are actively transported across the placenta to mineralize the fetal skeleton. Premature infants (<30 weeks) are particularly liable to develop rickets because:
1 Their postnatal intake of calcium and phosphorus is much less than they would have accrued *in utero*. This applies even when they are fully fed on breast milk or conventional formulae; breast milk is particularly low in phosphorus.
2 Prolonged intravenous feeding is also likely to lead to rickets because it is difficult to get sufficient phosphate into the commonly used solutions.
3 The dietary lack of phosphorus results in further bone demineralization to release phosphate required for many intracellular enzyme systems.
4 The infant may receive insufficient vitamin D; this, however, is easily overcome by supplementation (Chapter 13).

Diagnosis

1 The bones appear 'washed out' on X-ray, with rachitic splaying of bone ends.

Table 26.1. Features of some skeletal dysplasias presenting at birth.

Syndrome	Head	Chest	Bony features	Other features	Outcome
Achondrogenesis (AR)	Normal/large	Narrow	Micromelia + + + vertebrae and pelvis not ossified	Depressed nasal bridge	Lethal
Thanatophoric dwarfism (? inheritance)	Large	Narrow + + +	Short, bowed long bones	Large forehead, small facies, small foramen magnum	Lethal
Asphyxiating thoracic dystrophy (AR)	Normal	Narrow + + +	Short ribs + + +	Lung hypoplasia, cystic dysplastic, kidneys	Usually lethal but can survive
Achondroplasia (AR)	Large	Normal	Short tubular bones	Large forehead, depressed nasal bridge	Good, Normal IQ
Diastrophic dwarfism (AR)	Normal	Normal	Thick, short tubular bones, specially first metacarpal	Talipes, medial twisting of hands	Good Normal IQ

Camptomelic dysplasia (AR)	Normal	Narrow +++	Bent, long bones	Flat face, micrognathia, anti-mongoloid slant to eyes	Usually lethal, low IQ
Rhizomelic chondrodysplasia punctata (AR)	Normal/large	Normal	Short femora and humeri. Epiphyseal punctate calcification	Depressed nasal bridge +++, cataracts	Usually lethal, low IQ
Osteogenesis imperfecta (AR)	Normal/large	Normal	Multiple fractures, poorly mineralized bones	Short, bent limbs, depressed nasal bridge, bleeding tendency	Usually lethal — survivors have multiple fractures
Osteogenesis imperfecta (AD)	Normal	Normal	Thin, fractures in early life	Bowed, long bones, short sture	multiple fractures in early life — usually wheelchair-bound

NB AR = Autosomal recessive   AD = Autosomal dominant

2 Alkaline phosphatase levels may be greatly elevated (>1000 u/l).
3 The infant may be hypophosphataemic.

Prognosis

Such infants may suffer rib fractures resulting from the demineralization. Eventually the osteopenia improves over the course of many
months as dietary intake becomes adequate.

Treatment

1 Adequate vitamin D supplementation (p.107).
2 Adding phosphate supplements to breast milk.
3 Using special preterm formulae (p.108).
Prevention is by providing an adequate dietary intake of calcium and
phosphate.

Dwarfs

There are a number of syndromes of short-limbed dwarfism presenting at birth. All are individually very rare, some are rapidly lethal;
most have a hereditary basis and therefore correct diagnosis is essential for genetic counselling. Some of the salient features of the skeletal
dysplasias are listed in Table 26.1.

Osteogenesis imperfecta

There are various forms of this disease. The two types that may be
seen in neonates are:

Type I (AD) 10% of affected infants have intra-uterine fractures and
most will develop them before 5 years. Later manifestations include
severe orthopaedic deformities, blue sclerae and deafness.

Type II (AR) Multiple antenatal fractures; lethal.
      There are at least two other types which are not usually diagnosed
in the neonatal period. One has similar manifestations to the type I
with a later onset; the other is a very mild form and not diagnosed
until adult life. Both are autosomal dominant.

Congenital hypophosphatasia

This condition is lethal. The limbs are short and all bones are *grossly* undermineralized.

Further reading

Hensinger, R.N. (1981) *Neonatal Orthopedics*. Grune & Stratton, New York.

Chapter 27
Congenital Malformations

Chromosome abnormalities

Trisomies

The three commonest trisomic conditions, Trisomy 13 (Patau's syndrome), Trisomy 18 (Edward's syndrome) and Trisomy 21 (Down's syndrome) should all be recognized early in the neonatal period; their features are listed in Table 27.1. In every case the diagnosis should be confirmed by chromosome analysis to identify the small percentage of cases (circa 5%) due to translocation. Infants with trisomies 13 and 18 have lethal malformations which are incompatible with survival.

In the case of infants with Down's syndrome, great care should be taken to exclude congenital heart disease and gut malformations such as duodenal atresia and Hirschsprung's, which are more common in these infants. Their parents should always be informed of the diagnosis before discharge from the maternity hospital.

Turner's syndrome

Though often not recognized, this condition can be diagnosed in the neonatal period in female infants with a short neck, low hairline, widely-spaced nipples, congenital heart disease and oedema of the feet.

Sex chromosome abnormalities

Syndromes such as XXY, XXX, XYY are not usually recognizable in the neonatal period.

The child with multiple malformations

Always document the abnormalities very carefully; take photographs and X-rays if possible, and always do a chromosome analysis. Individual syndromes can then be recognized and appropriate genetic counselling given to the parents.

302

Table 27.1. The three commonest trisomic conditions.

	Trisomy 21	Trisomy 18	Trisomy 13
Incidence	1:600	1:2000	1:5000
General	Happy docile children; enjoy mimicry and listening to music	Feeble cry, premature or postmature	—
Growth	Small for dates	Small for dates	Small for dates
CNS	Slower than normal	Survival rare	Survival rare
	Hypotonia ++, IQ 25–50	Hypertonic	Holoprosencephaly; agenesis of corpus callosum, spina bifida, hypertonic, IQ ++ retarded
		IQ retarded ++	
Cranium	Flat occiput, third fontanelle, microcephaly	Prominent occiput, narrow bifrontal diameter, microcephaly	Wide fontanelle, hypertelorism, microcephaly
Eyes	Upward slanting eyes, squint, epicanthus, Brushfield's spots	Short palpebral fissure, epicanthus	Microphthalmia, coloboma, anophthalmia, cyclopia
Ears	Small, overlapping upper helices, low-set	Low-set and malformed	Low-set, odd helices, deaf
Nose	Small, low nasal bridge		
Mouth	Small maxilla and palate, fissured protruding tongue	Small, narrow, arched palate, micrognathia, cleft lip and palate	Hare lip, cleft palate, cleft tongue, micrognathia
Neck	Broad, short		

Table 27.1. (continued).

	Trisomy 21	Trisomy 18	Trisomy 13
Chest	—	Abnormal or absent right lung, short sternum, hypoplastic nipples	—
Hands	Short hands and fingers, single palmar crease, clinodactyly of fifth fingers, distal palmar triradius	Clenched with overlapping fingers, small nails, ulnar deflection of hand, small thumb	Overlapping fingers, distal triradius, hyperconvex nails, polydactyly, ulnar deflection, radial aplasia, syndactyly
Feet	Gap between first and second toes	Small hallux, TEV, rocker bottom feet	Rocker bottom feet, small nails and TEV
Gut/abdomen	Diastasis recti, duodenal atresia, TOF, Hirschsprung's	Umbilical hernia, diastasis recti, malformation of anus, Meckel's diverticulum	Omphalocele, umbilical hernia, malrotation
Skin	Dry	Redundant and hairy	Haemangiomata, scalp defects, loose neck skin
CVS	AV canal, VSD.	VSD, ASD	VSD, PDA, dextrocardia
Genitalia/renal	—	Hydronephrosis, polycystic kidneys, cryptorchid, small labia, horshoe kidney	Cryptorchid, odd scrotum, bicornuate uterus, hypospadias, polycystic kidneys, hydronephrosis
X-ray	Hypoplastic acetabula and flat acetabular and iliac angles, hypoplastic mid phalanx fifth finger	—	Pelvic hypoplasia, thin ribs

Table 27.2. Abnormal phenotypes and genotypes which are commonly encountered.

	Trisomy 8	Tripoidy	Cri-du-chat
Incidence	Rare	Rare	Rare
General	Usually mosaics	Most are neonatal deaths	Deletion 5p and cat-like cry
Growth	Moderately decreased	IUGR +++	IUGR+ and slow growth
CNS	IQ reduced ++	Brain malformation, hydrocephalus	Reduced IQ ++, hypoyonia++
Cranium	Prominent forehead, hypertelorism	Large posterior fontanelle	Microcephaly, hypertelorism
Eyes	Deep-set, squint	Microphthalmia, coloboma	Epicanthus, squint, down-sloping eyes
Ears	Prominent, cupped, thick helices	Low-set, malformed	Low-set, malformed
Nose/face	Prominent nares	—	Round face
Mouth	Full lips, high arched palate	—	Cleft lip/palate
Neck	—	—	—
Chest	—	—	—
Hands	Camptodactyly, deep grooves	Some syndactyly 3–4; simian crease	Distal triradius; simian crease
Feet	Grooved ++	TEV	—
Gut/abdomen	—	—	—
Skin	—	—	—
CVS	—	CHD (various)	CHD (various)
Genitalia	—	Hypospadias, cryptorchid	—
Renal	—	Cystic dysplasia	—
X-ray	—	—	—
Other	—	Small adrenals	—

Table 27.2. (continued).

	18p-Syndrome	18q-Syndrome	Cornelia de Lange
Incidence	Rare	Rare	Moderately rare
General	—	—	—
Growth	Moderately reduced	Moderately reduced	IUGR+ and delayed growth
CNS	Decreased IQ +, hypotonia	Marked reduction IQ, hypotonia, nystagmus	++ reduced IQ, hypertonic
Cranium	Mild microcephaly, hypertelorism	Microcephaly	Small, flat skull
Eyes	Ptosis, epicanthus	—	Bushy eyebrows, synophrys
Ears	Large, protruding	Deaf, big antihelix and antitragus	—
Nose/face	—	Mid-facial hypoplasia	Small nose with anteverted nostrils
Mouth	Wide mouth	Carp shaped, narrow palate	Thin lips, beak on upper lip, high arched palate, long philtrum
Neck	—	—	—
Chest	Pectus excavatum	—	—
Hands	Small	Long with tapering fingers, distal triradius, simian crease	Small with reduction deformities, simian crease
Feet	Small	TEV, funny toes	Small with reduction deformities
Gut/abdomen	—	—	—
Skin	—	—	Hairy, small nipples
CVS	—	—	—
Genitalia	—	Hypoplastic (both sexes)	Hypoplastic in male
Renal	—	—	—
X-ray	—	—	—
Other	Reduced IgA	—	—

Table 27.2. (continued).

	Prader–Willi	Zellweger	Moebius
Incidence	Moderately rare	Rare	Moderately rare
General	—	Cerebral-hepato-renal syndrome, peroxisomal disorder	—
Growth	IUGR	—	—
CNS	Hypotonia++, IQ 40–60	Hypotonia, fits, macrogyria, polymicrogyria	VI, VII, nerve palsies, occasionally others
Cranium	Narrow skull	Large fontanelle, flat occiput and face	—
Eyes	—	Epicanthus, Brushfield's spots, nystagmus	—
Ears	—	—	—
Nose/face	—	Flat face	Mask-like
Mouth	—	Micrognathia	Micrognathia
Neck	—	Redundant skin	—
Chest	—	—	—
Hands	Small	Simian crease	—
Feet	Small	TEV	—
Gut/abdomen	—	Hepatomegaly	—
Skin	—	—	—
CVS	—	PDA, VSD	—
Genitalia	Cryptorchid, hypogonadism	—	—
Renal	—	Cysts and albuminuria	—
X-ray	—	Stippled epiphyses	—
Other	Subsequent obesity	Limb contractures	—

Table 27.2. (continued).

	Rubinstein–Taybi	Hallerman–Streiff	Smith–Lemli–Opitz
Incidence	Moderately rare	Rare	Rare
General	—	—	—
Growth	Short stature plus reduced IQ	Small	IUGR+, reduced growth
CNS	—	—	Hypotonia ++, ++reduction in IQ
Cranium	Microcephaly	Flat head, prominent forehead	Microcephaly, narrow frontal area
Eyes	Down-slanting eyes, ptosis epicanthus, squint	Microphthalmia cataract	Ptosis, epicanthus, squint
Ears	Low set, malformed	—	Low-set, slanting
Nose/face	Hypoplastic maxilla, hooked nose	Small, thin pointed nose	Broad nasal tip, anteverted nostrils
Mouth	—	Small with high palate and poor teeth	Micrognathia, thick alveolar ridges
Neck	—	—	—
Chest	—	—	—
Hands	Broad thumbs with radial angulation	—	Simian crease
Feet	Broad hallux	—	Syndactyly 2–3
Gut/abdomen	—	—	—
Skin	—	Atrophic	—
CVS	—	—	—
Genitalia	Cryptorchism	—	Cryptochism, hypospadias
Renal	—	—	—
X-ray	—	—	—
Other	—	—	—

Table 27.2. (continued).

	Beckwith–Wiedemann	Meckel–Gruber	Treacher–Collins
Incidence	Moderately rare	Rare	Common
General	Large muscle mass, fat	—	—
Growth	Large	IUGR	—
CNS	If hypoglycaemic maybe reduced, otherwise normal IQ	Posterior encephalocele cerebellar hypoplasia, hydrocephaly	—
Cranium	Metopic ridge, prominent occiput	Microcephaly	
Eyes	Prominent	Microphthalmia	Antimongoloid slant, lower lid coloboma, absent eyelashes
Ears	Odd fissures on ear lobule	—	Malformed, rudimentary, deafness
Nose/face	—		
Mouth	Macroglossia ++	Micrognathia, cleft lip	Small jaw, cleft palate
Neck	—	Short, webbed	—
Chest	—	—	—
Hands	—	Polydactyly	—
Feet	—	Talipes	—
Gut/abdomen	Omphalocele, diastasis recti	—	—
Skin	—	—	—
CVS	—	CHD	—
Genitalia	—	Cryptorchid	—
Renal	Large kidneys (occasional Wilms' tumour)	Polycystic, hypoplastic	—
X-ray	—	—	—
Other	Hypoglycaemia with hyperinsulinism, polycythaemia	—	—

Table 27.2. (continued).

	Fetal alcohol	Fetal phenytoin	Goldenhar	Oro-facial-digital
Incidence	Uncertain	Uncertain	Rare	Moderately rare
General	—	—	—	X-linked dominant, lethal in males
Growth	IUGR and poor growth	Mild IUGR	—	—
CNS	Reduced IQ, clumsy	Reduction IQ ±	—	reduced IQ ±
Cranium	Microcephaly, short palpebral fissures	Big fontanelle, hypertelorism	—	—
Eyes	—	—	Epibulbar dermoid	—
Ears	—	Low-set	Small, rudimentary, deafness	—
Nose/face	Mid-facial hypoplasia	Depressed nasal bridge	—	Small nose
Mouth	Smooth philtrum	Broad alveolar ridge, cleft lip and palate	Small maxilla and mandible	Webbing between alveolous and buccal mucus membranes, clefts and ridges of lips, alveoli and tongue, anomalous teeth
Neck	—	Short	—	—
Chest	—	—	—	—
Hands	Small nails	Hypoplastic phalanges, very small nails	—	—
Feet	—	—	—	—
Gut/abdomen	—	—	Pre-auricular tags	—
Skin	Hirsutism	Coarse, hairy	—	—
CVS	—	—	—	—
Genitalia	—	—	—	—
Renal	—	—	—	—
X-ray	—	—	—	—
Others	Joint abnormalities	—	Hemivertebrae	—

Excellent catalogues of abnormal phenotypes and genotypes are provided in Smith (1982). In Table 27.2 we list some of those malformations which are more commonly encountered, and which can be recognized in the neonatal period.

Reference

Smith, D.M. (1982) *Recognisable Patterns of Human Malformation*, 3rd edn., W.B. Saunders Co., Philadelphia.

Further reading

Baraitser, M. & Winter, R.F. (1986) Congenital malformations. In *Textbook of Neonatology*, N.R.C. Roberton (ed.), Churchill Livingstone, Edinburgh, pp.495–526.

Chapter 28
Skin Problems in the Newborn

The neonate's skin may exhibit many transient rashes and 'birth marks'. Because it is relatively thin and delicate it is easily traumatized providing an entry for infection. Several rare inherited skin disorders appear in the neonatal period.

Common problems

Harlequin colour change

This is a dramatic transient colour change with one side of the baby pale and sharply demarcated from the other half, which is pink. It rapidly fades and is of no significance.

Milia

These yellow or white spots 1 mm in diameter over cheeks, nasal bridge and naso-labial folds are a normal finding in about 40% of neonates and mark the openings of sebaceous glands.

Milaria (sweat rash)

These 1–2 mm, superficial, non-inflammatory vesicles over forehead, neck and skin folds, may be induced by a warm environment and resolve on removal to a cool one.

Erythema toxicum (urticaria neonatorum)

This transient maculo-papular rash occurs in 30–70% of normal-term neonates (very rare in the preterm) with a peak incidence at 48–96 hours. The rash may become very dramatic; the papules appear white or yellow and are full of eosinophils. The rash may be mistaken for skin sepsis, but no treatment is required.

312

Pustular melanosis

This rare, benign and transient rash is present at birth (cf. erythema toxicum). It occurs mainly over the neck, back, forehead and shins and consists of small vesiculo-pustules that rupture within 24–48 hours, leaving a central hyperpigmented macule with a collar of scale. All types of lesion may be present together but the macules may persist for 3 months. The vesicles contain polymorphs and are sterile. It should not be mistaken for sepsis, or treated.

Nappy rash

This common erythematous eruption is frequently accompanied by maceration and scaling. It is usually caused by friction or irritation from excreta, but sometimes arises from contact with soaps and detergents. It generally responds to exposure and barrier creams. Plastic pants should be avoided. Monilial nappy rash, often associated with oral thrush, causes a vesicular eruption which becomes a confluent bright red macerated rash over the nappy area with satellite lesions outside it. Treatment is exposure and topical nystatin cream. Treat the oral thrush if present (p.172).

Seborrhoeic dermatitis

This is rare in the neonate. It consists of patchy red fissuring in skin folds with occasional weeping. After the neonatal period it is usually associated with thick greasy scales on the scalp (cradle cap) or there may be a generalized weeping, scaling rash resembling infantile eczema. Treatment is with hydrocortisone ointment.

Skin sepsis (see also p.172)

Bullous impetigo. This consists of large bullae filled with straw-coloured fluid which quickly rupture leaving a red denuded area; *staphylococcus aureus* is the culprit and flucloxacillin is indicated (p.172).

Toxic epidermal necrolysis (Ritter, Lyell, or scalded skin syndrome). This is a severe staphylococcal infection with generalized erythema followed by rapidly spreading bullae, the epidermis peels off in sheets leaving a scalded skin appearance. Fever and fluid loss through the denuded skin may be severe. Treatment is systemic flucloxacillin plus general supporting care (p.176).

Petechial skin rashes

Petechiae, if generalized, usually signify thrombocytopenia with or without infection, e.g. septicaemia (bacterial or viral) or congenital infection (CMV, rubella, Chapter 16).

Naevi and birthmarks

Mongolian spots

These are present in 90% of coloured or oriental races and consist of grey-blue pigmented areas 2−10 cm diameter chiefly over buttocks, flanks and shoulders.

Giant hairy naevus

This is a rare deeply-pigmented lesion which may be very extensive or even multiple. Some have hairs, others have a smooth, leathery appearance. This is one of the few naevi that require treatment because they may turn malignant.

Cafe-au-lait spots

These are rare in the neonate and are not significant unless there are more than six (consider neurofibromatosis).

Simple naevus (salmon patch, 'stork bite')

This is the commonest birth-mark. The pale pink, flat lesions occur on forehead, eyelids and back of neck. They fade with time.

Port wine stain (naevus flammeus)

These permanent, sharply circumscribed, reddish-purple lesions do not fade. Those lying over the trigeminal area may be associated with ipsilateral intracranial vascular malformation (Sturge−Weber syndrome) causing convulsions, hemiparesis and mental retardation.

Strawberry naevi

These are rare at birth, are commoner in females and in premature infants, can occur anywhere on the body and are often multiple. They start as a small, bright red macule which gradually enlarges over the next 6−9 months to form a raised 'strawberry'.

Cavernous haemangioma

These lesions lie deeper in the dermis and are less well-defined than the strawberry, they give a bluish discolouration to the overlying skin and may feel like a 'bag of worms'. Sometimes there are mixed strawberry and cavernous lesions.

The natural history of both types of angioma is to enlarge and then involute. Parents often need repeated reassurance. Very large ones, which may cause thrombocytopenia, may respond to systemic steroids.

Inherited skin conditions (that may be seen in the neonate)

Epidermolysis bullosa simplex (AD)

Blisters are present at birth but the tendency improves with time and the prognosis is good.

Epidermolysis bullosa letalis (AR)

This is very rare and consists of large erosions present at birth with further sheets of skin desquamating afterwards and involvement of mucous membranes. Death from secondary infection is the usual outcome.

Epidermolysis bullosa dystrophica (AR)

Blistering and erosions are present at birth with involvement of the mucous membranes. The lesions, being deeper in the epidermis, lead to severe scarring, with contractures.

Lamellar icthyosis (non-bullous congenital icthyosiform erythroderma)

This autosomal recessive disease may present in one of three forms:
1 Generalized erythroderma followed by desquamation and a parchment-like appearance.
2 'Collodion' baby: infant born with a very tight and thickened

stratum corneum resembling collodion. There may be severe ectropion. The membrane sheds leaving an erythematous skin, but the prognosis is good. Both 1 and 2 develop icthyosis later in life.

3 Harlequin fetus: this is an extreme form of the above in which the infant is born with grotesque horny plates over the entire body, contractures are severe and the prognosis is hopeless.

Epidermolytic hyperkeratosis (bullous congenital icthyosiform erythroderma)

The infant is born with widespread erythroderma, bullae and a dry, peeling skin which is prone to secondary infection. Later there is marked hyperkeratosis and scaling which persists throughout life.

X-linked icthyosis

This is occasionally seen at birth presenting with mild scaling over the whole body (except palms and soles).

Further reading

Solomon, L.N. & Esterly, N.B. (1973) *Neonatal Dermatology*. W.B. Saunders Co., Philadelphia.

Chapter 29
Miscellanea

Ophthalmic Problems

Retinopathy of prematurity (retrolental fibroplasia)

Retinopathy of prematurity (ROP) occurs mainly in infants less than 1.5 kg birthweight and less than 32 weeks GA, and the incidence increases as birthweight and gestation fall (Table 29.1).

The condition is due to the oxygen tension in the retinal arterial blood being too high. However, many infants who have had prolonged exposure to dangerously high retinal P_aO_2 values do not develop ROP, whereas transient exposure in others of similar gestation and birthweight causes severe retinal damage. The danger level for retinal P_aO_2 is not accurately known, but levels greater than 14−16 kPa must be avoided. Other factors such as extreme prematurity, the presence of adult haemoglobin after transfusion, or vitamin E deficiency may so increase the neonate's susceptibility that ROP develops within the normal P_aO_2 range of 8−12 kPa.

The retinal damage goes through two phases, first a proliferative and then a cicatricial. Minor degrees of proliferative change may be seen in many LBW infants, and in 80−100% of them it regresses completely; in others, more severe proliferative changes with haemorrhage result in scarring — the cicatricial stage — which may be severe enough to cause macular distortion, retinal detachment and blindness.

Treatment

Minimize the incidence of ROP by keeping the arterial P_aO_2 below 12 kPa — and it may need to be kept even lower in infants less than 26 weeks gestation.

Table 29.1. Incidence of retinopathy of prematurity (ROP)

Birthweight	Cicatricial ROP (%)	Blind (%)
<1.0 kg	30	8
1.0−1.5 kg	2.2	0.5

Some ophthalmologists recommend cryotherapy of the retina should the proliferative changes become so marked that progression to permanent cicatricial changes seem likely.

Buphthalmos

This is the neonatal form of glaucoma, and may be primary, or secondary to other eye disease such as congenital rubella. The infant usually has photophobia, blepharospasm and increased production of tears. The eye is enlarged, with a hazy cornea and an increased intra-ocular tension. Urgent surgical treatment is necessary.

Cataract

Cataracts are occasionally seen on routine examination of a neonate's eyes, or may be picked up if a more meticulous ophthalmic examination is carried out in an infant who has a positive family history or signs of a condition in which cataracts occur, such as galactosaemia or congenital rubella. Many cataracts are first recognized by the mother, who notices a white reflex in her baby's pupil when he has his eyes open during a feed.

With unilateral cataracts little is gained by early surgery, since the infant relies entirely on his good eye, and develops supression amblyopia in the affected eye. With bilateral cataract, extraction should be considered in early infancy if any useful vision is to be preserved.

Infants of drug addicted mothers

Babies of mothers who are narcotic addicts have multiple neonatal problems including an increased incidence of prematurity, SFD, birth asphyxia and congenital infection. They do, however, have a reduced incidence of RDS. In the neonatal period, usually in the first 4 days, the infants may develop withdrawal symptoms. They become very irritable and jittery and scream; 10–20% have seizures. They may vomit, and can become very dehydrated and acidotic.

These problems are mitigated, but not avoided, by converting the mother to methadone antenatally. Treatment for symptomatic infants is usually needed for at least 3 weeks, and is best given as reducing doses of opiates such as morphine rather than by simple sedation with diazepam, chlorpromazine or phenobarbitone.

As well as infants of narcotic abusers, babies of mothers who are taking or abusing anticonvulsants, psychotropics and sedatives may have similar, albeit milder, neonatal 'withdrawal' symptoms. The treatment is sedation. Infants of cocaine addicts seem to have surprisingly few problems.

Hydrops fetalis

There are many causes of this condition characterized by gross oedema, ascites and pleural and pericardial effusions (Table 29.2). As rhesus incompatibility has become much rarer, the other conditions have become relatively more important.

Attempt to resuscitate all hydropic infants, since some of the conditions are compatible with neurologically intact survival; in others it is important to establish a diagnosis to assist with genetic counselling, or the management of subsequent pregnancies.

Hydrops is usually due to one or more of three interrelated factors:
1 Anaemia.

Table 29.2. Causes of hydrops (after Etches, 1986).

Haemolytic disease of the newborn
  Rhesus, ABO, Kelly, Duffy
Fetal anaemia
  haemorrhage into mother, twin;
  α-thalassaemia, G6PD deficiency
Fetal cardiac disorders
  congenital heart disease
  arrhythmias
  A/V malformations
Congenital infection
  CMV, toxoplasmosis, syphilis, leptospirosis, Chagas', parvovirus
Placental anomalies
  chorionic, umbilical vein thrombosis,
  chorioangioma
Fetal lung malformation
  lymphangiectasia,
  adenomatoid malformation
Fetal renal disorders
  congenital nephrotic syndrome, renal dysplasia
Fetal GI tract abnormalities — atresias, hepatitis
Hypoalbuminaemia, or albumin polymerization
Maternal diabetes, toxaemia, anaemia
Achondroplasia and other short limb dwarfs
Fetal malignancy, e.g. neuroblastoma
Multiple malformations and chromosomal disorders
Idiopathic (50% of all cases)

2 Hypoalbuminaemia due to liver damage.
3 Heart failure due to anaemia, cardiac abnormality or high output state.

Immediate treatment should be:

1 IPPV from the moment of delivery to control pulmonary oedema and severe hypoxaemia which are virtually always present.
2 Insert umbilical venous and arterial catheters at once to monitor BP and CVP, and to obtain blood for:

  a Haemoglobin, WBC and differential, platelet count.
  b Coombs' test, blood group, bilirubin.
  c Blood gases.
  d Electrolytes and blood urea.
  e Serology for intra-uterine infectious disease.
  f Haemoglobin electrophoresis.
3 Take blood cultures and a full range of swabs.
4 Arrange a chest X-ray, and a plain X-ray of the abdomen.
5 Aspirate the peritoneal and pleural effusions, taking care to avoid puncturing an underlying viscus.
6 Give 5 mg of frusemide i.v., and consider digitalization.

If the PCV is less than 25% it should be raised at once by exchange transfusion with fresh, uncrossmatched 0 Rh -ve blood. After the exchange transfusion do other diagnostic tests that are indicated.

If the infant does not pass urine within 6−12 hours of birth, peritoneal dialysis may be indicated. However, the mortality is high in cases in which no obvious and treatable cause can be found, and in whom there is no early response to treatment.

Malignant disease

This is extremely rare in the neonate, with an incidence of 2−3: 100 000 live births, i.e. about 15−25 cases per annum in Britain. The conditions identified are shown in Table 29.3. Most of the solid tumours present as a space-occupying lesion.

Leukaemia usually presents with hepatosplenomegaly and skin infiltration, plus evidence of marrow disorder such as anaemia and thrombocytopenia.

The outcome for neuroblastoma, Wilms' tumour and teratoma is very good with appropriate surgery, radiotherapy and chemotherapy. Neonatal leukaemia is of the myelogenous type, and is usually fatal.

Table 29.3. Neonatal cancer notifications in Great Britain for children born in 1970−77 (after Broadbent, 1986).

Neuroblastoma	27
Leukaemia	17
Malignant teratoma	16
Sarcoma	13
Brain tumour	12
Wilms'	8
Hepatoblastoma	3
Other	5
	—
Total	101

References

Broadbent, V.A. (1986) Malignant disease in the neonate. In *Textbook of Neonatology*, N.R.C. Roberton (ed.), Churchill Livingstone, Edinburgh. pp.689−95.

Etches, P.C. (1986) Hydrops fetalis. In *Texbook of Neonatology*, N.R.C. Roberton (ed.), Churchill Livingstone, Edinburgh. pp.484−94.

Chapter 30
Discharge and Early Post Discharge Care of Sick and Preterm Babies

Discharging babies

A normal term baby does not need to be in hospital. Women are delivered in hospital as a tacit recognition of the fact that the 30−60 minutes on each side of delivery are the most dangerous time for both mother and baby during the whole pregnancy. If this period is complication-free, a well mother and baby can go home.

For a fullterm baby who was ill in the neonatal period and has recovered, as with any other paediatric inpatient, he should be discharged, and there is no point in extending his period in hospital just because he is a neonate.

For LBW babies, the following factors should be considered when planning their discharge:
1 Their weight.
2 Their feeding capabilities.
3 Their ability to sustain their body temperature in conventional room temperatures.
4 Some assessment of the home situation and the mother's capacity for caring for a LBW baby.
Of these four criteria, the second and the third are by far and away the most important. Far too much attention is geared to the first, and many babies are kept in hospital unnecessarily until they achieve some predetermined weight.

In our experience most LBW babies, by the time they reach 1.8−2.0 kg have fully recovered from any early neonatal illness, feed well and maintain their body temperature, and can therefore be discharged. Those who are SFD can be successfully and safely discharged when they weigh only 1.5−1.75 kg.

Support for the family after discharge

The responsibility of the NNU towards the sick or LBW infant does not end when the patient and his parents walk out of the door. Many parents have had to wait 2 months or more for their baby, and have had to watch the highly professional and dispassionate staff of the

NNU doing everything for their baby with skill and calmness. The parents have had limited opportunities to learn baby care, and although many mothers will have spent time, in some cases extremely long periods of time, in the mothers' accommodation on the unit, helping to care for their preterm infant, this is no substitute for having sole responsibility for their own baby at home or on a PNW.

Various schemes have been evolved for helping parents after discharge. Some units rely on the district midwife and the GP, others on the health visitor, whereas others have nursing staff specifically appointed for this role. The parents should be told that they can always phone or visit the NNU any hour of the day or night for advice.

Follow-up

Up to 10% of VLBW survivors have some neurological handicap (Chapter 31), however a large percentage of infants in an NNU have only mild or transient illness of a sort which, prima facie, is unlikely to cause any sequelae.

Neonates at high risk of sequelae, who should always be followed up carefully, include:

1 All infants weighing less than 1.5 kg at birth.
2 All infants who required respiratory support by CPAP or IPPV.
3 All infants known to have had an intracranial haemorrhage.
4 All infants who had neonatal meningitis.
5 All infants who had a septicaemia.
6 All infants who required surgery.
7 All infants who had convulsions.
8 All infants with symptomatic hypoglycaemia.
9 All infants who suffered birth asphyxia severe enough to require admission to the NNU.
10 All infants with known malformations including congenital heart disease and murmurs (infants who have defects requiring routine surgery, e.g. extra digits, undescended testes, hare lip etc., can be followed up by the appropriate surgical team).
11 Infants in whom there is serious doubt about the family's ability to cope.
12 Infants with documented metabolic errors, e.g. phenylketonuria, haemophilia.
13 Infants who had NEC, particularly those who had a resection.
14 Infants who had haemolytic disease of the newborn, irrespective of whether or not they required exchange transfusion.

15 Infants with renal problems, particularly infection.

16 Infants who have had a peak plasma bilirubin higher than 350 mmol/l.

While this seems to be a long list, it does in fact exclude the large number of infants above 1.5 kg who form the bulk of an NNU population, and are either completely asymptomatic, or suffered from mild and transient respiratory illness.

Ophthalmological follow-up

At some stage before discharge from the NNU, or shortly afterwards, babies at risk from ROP must have a full ophthalmological examination.

In view of the high risk of ROP in babies less than 1.0 kg birthweight, *all* such infants should be checked irrespective of whether they received supplementary oxygen or not. For infants with birthweights between 1.0 and 1.5 kg, only those who received supplementary oxygen need to be checked, and for those weighing between 1.5−2.0 kg at birth, ophthalmological assessment is only necessary for those who were very premature (less than 32 weeks gestation) or who were in high oxygen concentrations for many days.

Well baby care of the ex-preterm baby

Much of this subject is identical to that of the normal fullterm infant, but we would highlight three points:

Milestones

Babies achieve their social and motor milestones at a given time from conception — not from the moment of birth. A baby born 14 weeks early will therefore achieve his standard milestones 14 weeks late if calculated from his date of birth. Thus he will not smile, although entirely normal, till 4−5 months of age, nor walk till 17−18 months of age. Parents should be warned of this.

Vitamin and mineral supplements

All LBW babies (<2.0 kg) should receive ferrous sulphate 50 mg daily, Folic acid 5 mg weekly, and multivitamin drops 0.6 ml daily until they are at least 6 months old.

Immunization and vaccination

Preterm babies should have the routine immunization schedule. This should be started according to their chronological age from birth rather than their post-conceptional age. Pertussis is as great, if not a greater hazard to the 4 month-old survivor whose birthweight was 1.0 kg than it is to the 4 month-old who was the product of an entirely healthy, fullterm pregnancy.

Because the risks of pertussis vaccination in children already brain-damaged are not adequately evaluated, we omit this component of the triple vaccine in the following infants:

- All infants known to have had an intracerebral haemorrhage
- All infants who had neonatal seizures
- All infants who suffered from severe birth asphyxia
- All infants who had neonatal CNS infections
- All infants who had symptomatic neonatal hypoglycaemia
- All infants known to have CNS malformations

Chapter 31
Survival and Sequelae after Neonatal Care

Survival of LBW infants

With modern neonatal intensive care, survival is now the rule for non-malformed infants of 30 weeks' gestation or more, and more than 1.25 kg birthweight. Below this gestation and birthweight the mortality increases the smaller and less mature the infant. Survival below 600 g birthweight and at gestations less than 24 weeks is rare.

Table 31.1 shows the survival rate in LBW infants; the results are surprisingly homogeneous all over the world. Fig. 31.1 gives up-to-date information from the Cambridge unit.

Table 31.1. Average survival for non-malformed infants of low birthweight and short gestation.

Birthweight: % survival		Gestation: % survival	
0.5−0.75 kg	20−30	24, 25 weeks	15−30
0.75−1.0 kg	50−60	26, 27 weeks	50−60
1.00−1.25 kg	80−85	28, 29 weeks	80−90
>1.25 kg	≥95	≥30 weeks	≥95

Survival after RDS

Most infants who die at short gestation now die not from RDS, but from one of its complications — pneumothorax, chronic lung disease, sepsis and in particular periventricular haemorrhage (Table 2.4). The techniques of artificial ventilation are now so good that no infant over 750 g birthweight should die from respiratory failure alone in the neonatal period. The survival for infants with RDS are given in Table 31.2.

Survival of SFD infants

So long as they survive labour (p.100), and are not malformed, SFD infants should have an identical survival to normally-grown infants of the same gestation.

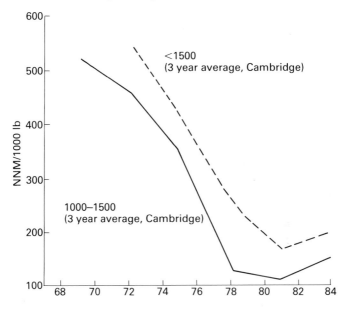

Fig. 31.1. Survival of VLBW infants.

Table 31.2. RDS incidence and outcome in Cambridge 1980−83.

Gestational age	Total births	Total RDS	Deaths from RDS plus complications
≤26 weeks	34	33	19
27−28 weeks	89	63	15
29−32 weeks	275	153	6
>32 weeks	11 719	93	0
Total	12 117	342 (2.8%)*	40 (12%)†

*Percentage of total births
†Percentage of total RDS

Neurological sequelae

Always remember two crucial facts about the epidemiology of handicap:
1 Of all severe handicap, only 10−15% arises in the perinatal period; even with cerebral palsy the figure is only 50%.
2 Of perinatally acquired handicap, including cerebral palsy, the majority arises in fullterm babies who suffer intrapartum asphyxia.

Neurological sequelae of birth asphyxia

Although severe birth asphyxia is now rare, (p.118), it is still an important cause of perinatally acquired handicap. Asphyxiated infants who had cerebral oedema, seizures and marked neurological abnormalities in the neonatal period often survive neurologically intact, but can have almost any neurological syndrome on follow-up, ranging from mild clumsiness and a slight reduction in IQ to severe mental retardation with microcephaly, spastic quadriplegia and sensory deficits.

There is some evidence that neonatal intensive care has reduced handicap from this source, but the responsibility for prevention lies primarily with the obstetrician since the brain damage in most of these babies arises pre-natally.

Neurological sequelae of LBW infants

For infants weighing more than 1.5 kg at birth compared with term infants there is little if any increased risk of neurological handicap in survivors, and when it does occur it is due primarily to intrapartum asphyxia. For infants between 1.0−1.5 kg, about 5% of survivors have a serious handicap, and a further 5% have an identifiable handicap — hemiparesis, diplegia or some hearing loss — which, however, is not serious enough to compromise their ability to be free-living, wage-earning, marrying, reproducing members of society. For infants less than 1.0 kg birthweight, the figures for serious and mild handicap may be double those for infants of 1.0−1.5 kg birthweight. In infants less than 1.0 kg birthweight, visual impairment from ROP is a major component of handicap in survivors.

In all survivors less than 1.5 kg, the presence or absence of a large PVH, particularly in association with PVL (p.219), is the major determinant of handicap (Table 31.3).

Evidence at present available suggests that the absolute numbers of VLBW infants surviving with handicap is remaining very constant and consists of about 5−10% of all VLBW babies delivered. However, as can be seen from Fig. 31.2, since the *absolute* numbers of VLBW infants who survive is increasing, the *proportion* of the survivors who are handicapped is falling. The fact that the percentage of surviving infants with birthweights of less than 1.0 kg who are handicapped is higher than that for infants weighing 1.0−1.5 kg is merely an indication of the lower survival rate under 1.0 kg.

Table 31.3. Outcome by severity of IVH ≤32 weeks' gestation (Stewart *et al.*, 1983).

CNS status on ultrasound	Total	Major abnormality (%)	
Normal	62	2	(3.2%)
Uncomplicated IVH	25	1	(4%)
Ventricular dilatation (8 transient, 4 hydrocephalus)	12	3	(25%)
Cerebral atrophy (± PVH grade IV)	9	6	(66%)

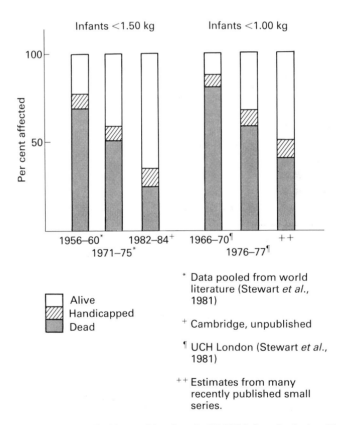

Fig. 31.2. Survival and incidence of handicap in VLBW infants in the last 30 years.

Neurological sequelae in SFD infants

Providing they have not suffered from severe birth asphyxia or symp-tomatic hypoglycaemia — both of which increase the risk of subse-quent CNS handicap — SFD neonates are no more prone to *severe* handicap than normally grown infants.

However, several studies have shown that compared with either normally grown infants of the same gestation, or infants of shorter gestations but similar birthweight, SFD infants consistently have an IQ which is about 5−10 points lower. The SFD infants with the lower IQ values are often those in whom there was ultrasonic evidence of reduced fetal head growth from the second trimester onwards, and in whom the lower IQ presumably represents reduced brain growth.

Developmental sequelae

Some VLBW survivors underachieve at school for their measured IQ, and have behaviour and learning difficulties. Whether this is a result of perinatally acquired organic brain damage, or whether it is due to prolonged neonatal mother-infant separation and the subsequent prob-lems with parenting, or is yet another manifestation of the poor socio-economic background from which most preterm babies arise, and to which they subsequently return, or whether, as seems most likely, it is a mixture of all three, remains speculative.

Non-neurological sequelae

Respiratory

Infants who suffered from neonatal pulmonary disease have an in-creased susceptibility to serious chest infections within the first 1−2 years. This is most marked in infants who were ventilated, and is almost universal in those who developed BPD (p.157).

Hospital admission

Very low birthweight survivors also have a higher admission rate to hospital within the first year of life for a multitude of conditions (Table 31.4), ranging from the increased incidence of inguinal hernia in VLBW males to continuing surgical procedures on infants who have colostomies for neonatal NEC, or shunts for hydrocephalus.

Table 31.4. First year morbidity requiring hospital admission in 90 survivors weighing <1.5 kg at birth (Hack *et al.*, 1981).

Infectious disease (mainly respiratory)	11
Inguinal herniorrhaphy	10
Ileostomy closure post NEC.	3
Failure to thrive	3
Post tracheostomy	2
Ligation of PDA	1
Near miss cot death	1
Broken arm (accidental)	1
Total	32

Cot death

The incidence of cot death is much higher in LBW survivors (Table 31.5).

Table 31.5. Incidence of cot death in infants of different gestations.

GA	Incidence/1000 LB
≤33 weeks	7.34
34–36 weeks	6.52
37–39 weeks	1.80
≥40 weeks	1.90

References

Hack, M., DeMonterice, D., Merkatz, I.R., Jones, P. & Fanaroff, A.A. (1981) Rehospitalisation of the very low birthweight infant. *American Journal of Diseases of Children* 135, 263–66.

Stewart, A.L., Reynolds, E.O.R. & Lipscombe, A.P. (1981) Outcome for infants of very low birthweight: Survey of the world literature. *Lancet* 1981 i, 1038–40.

Stewart, A.L., Thorburn, R.J., Hope, P.L., Goldsmith, M., Lipscombe, A.P. & Reynolds, E.O.R. (1983) Ultrasound appearance of the brain in very preterm infants and neurodevelopmental outcome at eighteen months of age. *Archives of Disease in Childhood* 58, 598–604.

Section VI

Chapter 32
Care of the Dying Baby and of the Parents After Perinatal Death

Perhaps because of the natural reticence of the medical profession about the death of one of their patients, this subject has not only been neglected in textbooks, but is often a neglected aspect of the care given in the NNU.

Irrespective of the circumstances, be the mother single or married, primiparous or multiparous, be the child a stillbirth or a neonatal death, be the pregnancy planned or unplanned, be the infant mal-formed — and perhaps therefore considered better dead — or nor-mally-formed, or be the death sudden and apparently unexplained, or a slowly losing battle against severe multisystem neonatal illness, the parents will always grieve for their dead baby. This grief will often be compounded in both parents by a feeling of guilt that they have failed not only themselves but their family and their spouse in the expected goal of producing a healthy, normal bouncing child or grandchild.

Too often in the past, it has been assumed that parents get over a perinatal death quickly, whereas more recently it has been recognized that grief in all its manifestations may last for at least a year or more, and must be allowed to run its course. The concept of the replacement baby — 'go out and have another one as soon as possible' is a disaster.

Care of the dying baby

Parents should always be kept fully informed about the medical progress of their ill baby, and once the prognosis is hopeless it should always be explained fully to them. As always, they, and other close relatives including siblings, should be allowed unrestricted access to the unit. If the death is not the result of a sudden deterioration and collapse, but is inevitable because of, for example, a huge intracerebral bleed, disseminated sepsis, irremediable hypotension, or brain death following severe intrapartum asphyxia, the baby should be discon-nected from the paraphernalia of intensive care and placed in an incubator or cot, if possible, in a separate room with his parents so that they can all be together in peace at the moment of death. The parents should be encouraged to hold and cuddle their dying and dead baby. Appropriate religous ceremonies should be arranged if requested.

Care of the lethally malformed baby

Infants with large and inoperable neural tube defects, Trisomy 13 and 18, Potter's syndrome, and other major malformations incompatible with long-term survival may live for days or weeks after birth. As with all other situations described in this chapter, the parents should be allowed to be as involved with their baby as they wish. Knowing that the outlook is hopeless, they may well choose to take their dying baby home and allow him to die there as a member of the family rather than have him die in an impersonal hospital setting. This should always be allowed, arranging to see them regularly on the ward or in outpatients, giving them 24-hour access to the paediatric department should a crisis arise which they feel unable to cope with at home.

Care of the parents after the death

The parents will, of course, have to endure the distressing routine of registering, often simultaneously, not only the birth but the death of their baby. The hospital can arrange to dispose of the bodies of the neonatal deaths, usually in an unmarked grave at a time that is convenient for the local undertaker when several bodies need to be interred. However parents can, and should, be encouraged to have a normal funeral even for babies of very short gestations, bearing in mind the exorbitant charges now made by undertakers.

In most cases a post-mortem should be carried out, not only to establish the precise cause of death, but also to check that nothing unsuspected is present which might influence the outcome of subsequent pregnancies. It will also tell the neonatologist whether anything which should have been done was left undone, or whether there were iatrogenic factors in the baby's demise. This practice is one of the most important components of what might be called 'quality-control' in neonatal intensive care.

Stillbirths

In the past, one of the things women who delivered stillbirths regretted most was that they were never allowed to see their baby and, as a result, had bizarre fantasies about what was wrong, and what he might have looked like.

The mother who has had an intra-uterine death has known the baby as a living being inside her, and needs to hold him and see him as part of her grieving. Therefore, parents should be allowed, and often actively encouraged, to see and hold their dead baby. This also applies to those whose stillborn child is malformed. Even anencephalics can be wrapped up in a blanket so that the face can be seen and the shock of seeing the whole malformation minimized.

Stillbirths are registered with a stillbirth cerificate, which the parents collect from the hospital, and have to lodge with the local registrar. They are now allowed to give the baby a Christian name. Although in many hospitals, stillborn babies are disposed of usually by burial in an unmarked plot in the local cemetery, the parents should always be asked whether they wish to arrange a conventional funeral, though in Britain they are unable to obtain the death grant for this. Stillbirths of less than 28 weeks gestation do not need a certificate, but an undertaker will arrange a funeral given a letter from the paediatrician explaining the situation.

If possible, all stillbirths should have a full post-mortem examination which should include a chromosome analysis, since chromosome anomalies are present in 5-10% of cases.

Subsequent counselling and care of the bereaved family

The obstetrician who has cared for the mother during her pregnancy producing a stillbirth, and the neonatologist who cared for the neonatal death should always see the parents some time after the death, preferably after the post-mortem results are available. They should discuss with the parents the cause of the baby's death in the light of the post-mortem findings, and in particular, they should try to assuage any guilt feelings which the parents may have. Appropriate counselling about subsequent pregnancies may be necessary if an inherited or recurring problem has been identified. More than one visit may be necessary for counselling; referral to a geneticist may be appropriate. The family GP must, of course, always be intimately involved.

Further reading

Forrest, G.C. (1983) Mourning Perinatal Death. In *Parent Baby Attachment in Premature Infants*, J.A. Davis, M.P.M. Richards, N.R.C. Roberton (eds), Croom Helm, Beckenham. pp.200-10.

Section VII

Chapter 33
Procedures

Taking blood

Capillary samples

These are generally used when only small quantities of blood are needed, e.g. Guthrie tests, Dextrostix or blood sugar, bilirubin, PCV and blood counts. In fact capillary blood can be used for most biochemical tests if the laboratory can provide suitable ultra-micro analytical methods.

Technique

Use the sides of the heel avoiding the plantar aspect, otherwise tissue atrophy, painful inclusion dermoids and osteomyelitis of the calcaneum may develop. If the circulation is not good or the foot is cold, rub it or warm it to obtain an adequate blood flow. Sterilize the skin and preferably use an automatic lancet (e.g. 'autolet') which is much less painful than a standard one. Try to avoid having to squeeze the heel too much.

Capillary blood gases (pH. P_{CO_2}, base deficit. NB, not P_aO_2)

The results are only valid under the following circumstances:
1 After the first day of life.
2 With adequate peripheral circulation.
3 When the heel has been pre-warmed in water at about 40°C.
4 When there is a free flow of blood into the capillary tube with no air bubbles.

Venous samples

One of the easiest ways to take blood from a neonate is to insert a 21 FG needle without a syringe into a vein on the dorsum of the hand while holding the wrist and fingers in extreme palmar flexion; breaking the hub off the needle before insertion makes this even easier.

Once the needle is in the vein, the specimen tubes are simply held to catch the blood which drips out; the flow can be encouraged by alternately squeezing and relaxing the the grip on the hand. This method can be used for blood cultures by dripping the blood into the barrel of a syringe. Standard venepunctures can be performed on any superficial veins, usually the antecubital ones or occasionally the external jugular. Avoid femoral vein punctures (see below).

Arterial access

This may be with an umbilical arterial catheter (see below), a peripheral cannula or by arterial stab. If serial samples are anticipated it is wise to insert an arterial line, whereas if only a few samples are likely then intermittent arterial stabs are satisfactory. Remember, however, that painful stabs may dramatically lower the P_aO_2 at the time of sampling.

The radial, dorsalis pedis and posterior tibial arteries may be cannulated or used for punctures; they can often be visualized with a fibreoptic light source. Do not catheterize the brachial, temporal or femoral arteries, although the first two may be used for stabs; avoid the femoral if at all possible (danger of infecting the hip joint). If using the radial artery always confirm the presence of an ulnar artery by palpation or by demonstrating hand perfusion while occluding the radial pulse.

Intravenous infusions

Any superficial vein can be used; the most popular are those on the hand, forearm, antecubital fossa, foot, ankle, or scalp. Teflon cannulae (22 FG) can often be inserted and probably stay in place longer than the alternative 'butterfly' needles; the latter are often used for scalp vein drips particularly when only a short infusion is needed, e.g. blood transfusion.

Umbilical vessel catheterization

The umbilical arteries can be catheterized for several days after birth and the umbilical vein remains patent for much longer. The procedure should be done with sterile precautions. If catheterization is performed on the first day a ligature should be placed round the base of the cord before cutting it, so as to control any haemorrhage. Cut the stump about 1 cm from the skin margin; the vein is patulous and lies superiorly, the arteries are white and tortuous and are about 2–3 mm in diameter.

Umbilical artery catheter (UAC)

Hold the orifice of one of the arteries with fine forceps and tease it open with a dilator or iris forceps. Introduce the 4.0–5.0 FG catheter (pre-filled with heparinized saline) and advance it while simultaneously pulling the umbilical stump towards the infant's head. Secure the catheter by tying a purse string suture round the umbilical stump and then use several loops tied tightly round the catheter itself. Always check the position by X-ray, remembering that the artery passes down into the iliac fossa before reaching the aorta, and that the latter lies to the left of the mid-line. Do not leave the tip of the catheter opposite D12–L2 where the renal and coeliac arteries originate. The catheter should always be infused with a solution containing heparin (2 u/ml). These catheters can be left in place for several days or weeks.

Umbilical venous catheter (UVC)

The principal uses for a UVC are:
1 For exchange transfusions.
2 As an emergency venous line.
3 For central venous pressure measurements.
Preparation is as for a UAC. Insert a 4–6 FG saline-filled catheter until a good blood flow can be obtained. On the first day of life there is a good chance that the catheter will pass through the ductus venosus into the inferior vena cava; after this time it is likely to stay in the portal vein.

Thoracentesis

In an emergency a 21 FG butterfly needle attached to a syringe can be inserted into the second or third intercostal space anteriorly just outside the nipple line.

Chest drain

Use a FG 10 or 12 tube with an end hole and at least two side holes, aim to insert the drain into the third or fourth intercostal space in the mid-axillary line. Infiltrate the skin with local anaesthetic unless the infant is *in extremis*. Make a small nick in the skin, push the tube in with forceps, or use a disposable trocar in the tube, and always put a clamp across the tube to prevent it going in too far. Try to angle the tube anteriorly. Connect the tube to underwater drainage and apply suction at $10-15$ cmH$_2$O. Stitch in place making sure that there is no leak round the tube. Always check tube position and the success of the procedure by an X-ray (p.156).

Lumbar puncture

This is usually an easier procedure in neonates than adults; it can be done in the lateral or sitting position. Use a 21 or 22 FG LP needle or a 21 FG butterfly. Aim for the L 3−4 space and advance the needle very slowly; the subarachnoid space is only $0.5-1$ cm from the skin surface.

Suprapubic aspiration

Use a 21 FG needle on a syringe, insert it in the mid-line just above the symphysis pubis and angle it slightly towards the pelvis; the bladder is entered at about 2 cm from the surface.

Appendix
Normal Values

The data in this section are drawn from a large number of sources in the neonatal and paediatric literature. In many cases the tables presented are a composite of what has been published elsewhere, and no references are therefore given.

Table A1. Normal biochemical values in the newborn.

Alanine aminotransferase	9−44 u/l at 37°C
Albumin	29−55 g/l
Alkaline phosphatase	125−575 u/l at 37°C
Ammonia	34−107 μmol/l
Aspartate aminotransferase (SGOT)	20−74 u/l at 37°C
Copper	2.7−9.3 μmol/l
Cortisol	330−1700 nmol/l
Folic acid	5−21 ng/ml
17-hydroxyprogesterone	<30 mmol/l (2−7 days)
	<14 mmol/l (>6 days)
IgG	630−1700 mg/100 ml
IgA	<8 mg/100 ml
IgM	<20 mg/100 ml
Insulin	2−20 μmol/ml
17 ketosteroids	<2.5 mg/24 hours
Osmolality	260−300 mmol/kgH$_2$O
Pregnanetriol	<0.2 mg/24 hours
TSH	<10 μmol/ml after 3 days
T4	75−350 nmol/l
T3	0.8−5.0 nmol/l
Zinc	10.7−15.6 μmol/l

Table A2. Normal blood electrolyte and urea values.

	Na (mmol/l)	K (mmol/l)	Ca (mmol/l)	PO$_4$ (mmol/l)	Urea (mmol/l)	Creatinine (μmol/l)
Premature newborn	132–140	4.5–7.2	1.90–2.80	1.1–2.6	1.5–6.7	55–150
Fullterm	130–145	3.6–5.7	2.10–2.70	1.8–3.0	1.6–4.6	35–115
1 week	–	4.0–6.4	2.20–2.75	1.39–3.03	1.6–4.2	14–86
1 month	–	4.0–6.2	2.15–2.95	1.29–3.04	1.9–5.2	12–48
Child	136–145	3.3–4.7	2.5–3.0	1.29–1.78	3.3–6.6	30–81

Table A3. Normal urine biochemistry.

Ca	0.2−1.6 mmol/l	0.06−0.21 mmol/kg/24 hours
Phosphate	<10 mmol/l	5−25 mmol/kg/24 hours
Na	1−15 mmol/l	0.15−2.2 mmol/kg/24 hours
K	2−28 mmol/l	0.2−1.2 mmol/kg/24 hours
Cl	5−30 mmol/l	1.3−3.3 mmol/kg/24 hours
Creatinine clearance	15−25 ml/minute/1.73^2 in premature infants <1 week 20−45 ml/minute/1.73^2 in fullterm infants	
Urea	2.5−4.5 mmol/24 hours	1.3−5.9 mmol/kg/24 hours

Table A4. Normal leucocyte counts in the first month of life.

Age	Neutrophils	Lymphocytes
24 hours	5.0−21.0	2.0−11.5
1 week	1.5−10.0	2.0−17.0
1 month	1.0−9.0	2.5−16.5

Table A5. Normal red cell values during the first week of life in the term infant.

	Day 1	Day 7
Haemoglobin (g/dl)	18.4	17.0
Packed cell volume (PCV)	0.58	0.54
Red cell count ($\times 10^{12}$/l)	5.8	5.2
Mean corpuscular volume (MCV fl)	108	98.0
Mean corpuscular haemoglobin concentration (MCHC g/dl)	32	33
Mean corpuscular haemoglobin (MCH pg)	35	32.5

Table A6. ECG standards (neonatal period); values relating to term neonates.

		QRS Axis	P.II	R.V₁ mv	R.V₅ mv	R.V.₆ mv	S.V₁ mv	S.V₆ mv
	95%	+185°		2.35	1.8	1.0	1.8	0.8
0.1 days	50%	+135°		1.3	1.0	0.4	0.8	0.3
	5%	+90°		0.7	0.3	0.1	0.1	0.0
	95%	+185°		2.4	1.9	1.0	1.8	0.75
1−3 days	50%	+135°		1.5	1.1	0.4	0.8	0.3
	5%	+90°		0.7	0.4	0.1	0.1	0.0
	95%	+180°		2.1	1.9	1.1	1.5	0.8
3−7 days	50%	+135°		1.25	1.3	0.5	0.7	0.3
	5%	+90°		0.5	0.5	0.15	0.1	0.0
	95%	+150°		1.7	2.1	1.3	1.0	0.8
7−30 days	50%	+110°		1.0	1.4	0.5	0.4	0.3
	5%	+75°		0.4	0.6	0.25	0.1	0.0

Table A7. Simplified criteria for diagnosing ventricular hypertrophy in the neonatal period.

	1−7 days	After 7 days
Right ventricular hypertrophy	qR pattern in V₁ *or* Total absence of both Q and S in V₁ (i.e. monophasic R) *or* R>28 mm in V₁ S> 14 mm in V₆	R>20 mm in V₁ S>10 mm in V₆ *or* Positive T in V₁
Left ventricular hypertrophy	RV₆>15 mm	RV₆>20 mm
Biventricular hypertrophy	Evidence of LVH and RVH or R+S in V₂ or V₃ or V₄>55 mm	

Table A8. Normal birthweights for Caucasian newborn (it is a matter of clinical judgement whether smallness for dates is taken as babies weighing below the fifth centile, or more than two standard deviations below the mean).

	−2SD	5th centile	Average	+2SD
22	280	—	485	690
23	350	—	580	810
24	450	—	660	865
25	610	—	825	1030
26	620	—	910	1200
27	670	—	1020	1370
28	660	550	1160	1680
29	750	740	1300	1870
30	800	790	1450	2140
31	960	990	1685	2330
32	1135	1100	1840	2525
33	1255	1365	2065	2790
34	1435	1740	2250	3040
35	1580	1855	2485	3370
36	1840	2085	2740	3640
37	2090	2270	2960	3845
38	2325	2450	3170	4035
39	2490	2580	3340	4230
40	2600	2685	3450	4350
41	2650	2745	3535	4460
42	2665	2760	3560	4470
43	2525	2730	3500	4500
44	2470	2670	3465	4460

Index

Page references in *italic* indicate figures and/or tables